1-15

MAD CHURCH DISEASE

HEALING FROM CHURCH BURNOUT

by

Anne Marie Miller

Expanded Fifth Anniversary Edition

Praise for Mad Church Disease

Anne Marie Miller has taken the problem by the jugular and brings remedy. Infused with a lively and informative style, Mad Church Disease is a life-saving resource for anyone in ministry—vocational or volunteer—who would like to understand, prevent, or treat the epidemic of burnout in church culture.

> — Dr. Wayne Cordeiro, senior pastor, New Hope Christian Fellowship, Honolulu, Hawaii, and author of The Divine Mentor

Anne Marie Miller is the real deal. And I appreciate her honest approach to a touchy topic. Mad Church Disease is a must-read for anyone who has gotten burned or burned-out by the church.

> — Mark Batterson, lead pastor, National Community Church, Washington, D.C., and author of Wild Goose Chase

This oft-ignored disease of the church is compromising the overall health of the American church. We've all had a touch of it—some have succumbed to it. This book hits the nail on the head clearly and does so with hope. Every minister should read Mad Church Disease—not just once, but from time to time.

> — Bob Roberts Jr., senior pastor, NorthWood Church, Keller, Texas, and author of The Multiplying Church

Every Christian leader intends to "finish our race well." Yet far too many of us end up escaping into sin or becoming numb, embittered, and angry. Mad Church Disease offers all of us the hope that we can actually make it to the end of the race, loving God and others with greater passion and being filled with audacious joy. Anne Marie Miller writes with raw honesty and hard-earned wisdom from her own story of burnout.

> — Nancy Beach, teaching pastor, Willow Creek Community Church, South Barrington, Illinois, and author of Gifted to Lead

My first thought: "What does a twenty-eight-year-old know about burnout?" Then I read this story about a girl named Anne, who grew up in a pastor's home and has lived through enough experiences to know what she's talking about. Anne Marie Miller not only tells her own story, but she gracefully integrates principles that have me at times saying, "That's right!" and at other times admitting, "That's me." As soon as I can, I'll be ordering enough copies for our entire staff.

— Tim Stevens, executive pastor, Granger Community Church, Granger, Indiana, and author of Pop Goes the Church

From the perspective of her own devastating personal experience, as well as by means of strongly researched facts, Anne Marie Miller opens our eyes to the crisis of ministry burnout. This paralyzing and contagious condition has wounded so many in church leadership. Mad Church Disease is a light on the path to healing and health.

— Nancy Ortberg, author of Unleashing the Power of Rubber Bands

I cannot say enough about how important the ideas put forth in Mad Church Disease are. With refreshing humility, grace, and transparency, Anne Marie Miller reveals the realities of burnout and how we can avoid being infected by this vicious disease. If you truly want to thrive and survive in ministry, this book is a must-read.

— Mike Foster, founder of People of the Second Chance

Burned-out leaders are heading up the mass exodus out of the inherited church. Anne Marie Miller's book Mad Church Disease brings much-needed attention to the dark compulsions of celebrity-driven churches that abuse and spew out our best people. But it does more than that. It also offers hope through stories of survival, pertinent scriptural teaching, and the prescription of a balanced, healthy, holistic lifestyle that will ensure longevity and the kind of joyful service that leaves no casualties. I wish I had read this book ten years ago. My family wishes I had read it twenty years ago!

— Andrew Jones, blogger at Tall Skinny Kiwi, tallskinnykiwi.typepad.com

Mad Church Disease

Copyright © 2009, 2014 by Anne Marie Miller

Requests for information should be addressed to:

anne@annemariemiller.com

Library of Congress Cataloging-in-Publication Data
  Miller, Anne Marie, 1980 –
    Mad church disease : healing from church burnout / Anne Marie Miller.
      p. cm.
    Includes bibliographical references.
    ISBN 978-0-9913735-3-6(paperback)
    1. Burn out (Psychology) — Religious aspects — Christianity.

Printed in the United States of America

08 09 10 11 12 13 14 • 22 21 20 19 18 17 16 15 14 13 12 11 10 9 8
7 6 5 4 3 2 1

"Never give up on church."

I leaned in close to his face as my grandfather whispered those words hours before he passed away.

Those were the last five words he spoke to me.

At the time, I had no idea the weight those words would someday carry.

This book is dedicated to you, Grandpa Emmett.

And I promise I won't.

The stories in this book are true. When needed, those named or those who are able to represent them gave me permission to use their stories.

For those who were unavailable to contact, irrelevant details of the anecdotes and names have been changed to respect their identities.

I am not a doctor, and the content in this book does not constitute medical or psychological advice.

Where necessary, please use your best judgment and consult medical professionals when embarking on your journey to health.

May the peace of Christ be with you and with your spirit,

Anne Marie Miller

Contents

Part 4: Practical Steps for Healthy Ministry

Part 5: Creating a Healthy Environment

Foreword

Years ago, during a particularly low time in my life and ministry, I sat in a leadership conference hoping for something — anything — that would relieve the pain I felt so deeply.

I loved Jesus, but his church was wearing me out.

One of my ministry heroes, Bill Hybels, took the stage. As usual, I was mesmerized by his wisdom, passion, and authenticity. Without my ever seeing it coming, God blindsided me with some of Bill's words. I'll never forget the chills that shot down my spine the moment Bill explained his dilemma. Through sincere pain and an obvious desire to change, Bill openly confessed that "the way I was doing the work of God was destroying the work of God in my life."

That was it. Someone had finally put words to what I felt so deeply. The way I was doing the work of God was destroying the work of God in me. Something had to change.

Why is it that the ones who are called to minister to others are often so dysfunctional? Why is it that those who help others heal are often so sick? Why is Jesus so loving and his church so difficult?

This week I had a conversation with a close pastor-friend. He confided in me the story that I've heard from ministers way too many times. He is miserable, hurting, exhausted, depleted — and flirting with spiritual burnout.

I've been praying for him for a long time. I am asking God that he keep my gifted friend from becoming another statistic — another broken pastor who crawls away from the church and his "calling," simply trying to survive and rebuild his life.

Something is wrong with the way many ministers minister.

Thankfully, in Mad Church Disease, Anne has courageously exposed her story, hurts, fears, and disappointments. This candid, humorous book will have you laughing, crying, groaning — and ultimately healing.

I am genuinely excited that you are reading this book. Or more accurately, that this book might be reading you. If you are a wounded spiritual warrior, I believe that God will use Anne's story and wisdom to initiate healing in your life. If you are a young and hungry minister, it will empower you to avoid many of ministry's dangerous land mines.

No matter what your context, your time in the exam room is approaching. God might diagnose you with a common ministry illness called "mad church disease." The great news is that he will bring healing through the book you hold in your hands.

— Craig Groeschel, founding and senior pastor, LifeChurch.tv

How to Use This Book

Use the study guide and additional resources available to you. You can find everything you need at ChurchBurnout.com.

Also, as anyone will tell you, always ask for a second opinion. I've made that part easy by including interviews I've done with leaders who I deeply respect. You'll gain wisdom from their thoughts about and experiences of burnout.

Author's Note

This book originally was published in February 2009. In February 2013, I got the news that it was "no longer financially feasible to print." Because I get emails on a weekly basis on the topic of burnout, I knew having this book out of print wasn't an option. So, after a year of trying my hand at self-publishing, and adding and updating pieces of this book (life experience, technology and such), here we are again.

Most of the content remains the same: it's a good message I strongly believe in. But I've edited a great deal and included five new chapters as well as produced some ancillary material like *Beating Burnout: A 30 Day Guide to Hope and Health* as well as some other resources that will constantly be changing and updating that you can find on ChurchBurnout.com.

Whether this is the first time you've owned this book or the fifth time you've read it, I pray it shows you that the only sacrifice required of you is your heart to God's. That is the only thing that truly matters and the separation between you and God has been taken care of on a cross.

Prologue: No Pity Parties Here

Growing up, pity parties were a specialty of mine. If my younger brother got a bigger present than I got at Christmas or if I didn't get cast as the lead in my school play, I would get down on myself. I'd lock myself in my bedroom and cry and cry and cry.

"Why me?"

When we run into obstacles we don't expect in life, it's easy to end up in that "Why me?" state of mind. It's extremely tempting to focus on the negative. After all, it isn't fair. It isn't what we had planned, and it screws everything up – or so it seems.

I've heard thousands of stories from people who have been hurt by the church. People who have given so much and asked for so little in return. They run and run and run until they collapse. Staff members, families, and volunteers. Men, women, and even children. The pain doesn't discriminate with regard to position, gender, or age.

And it's not fair.

And it does hurt.

There's a painful side to burnout we're not going to ignore.

However, locking ourselves in a figurative bedroom and focusing on all that's wrong in this world isn't going to do us — or the people who are entrusted to us — any good.

We've got to face the future

    with courage, hope, grace, and love —

        regardless of our circumstances.

We have to heal.

We have to be healthy.

I hope that together we will be able to align health and responsibility in a way that will illuminate the power and glory of the One who created us.

PART 1

HOW THE BURNOUT EPIDEMIC
IS KILLING THE GREATEST CALL

Chapter 1: The Preacher's Kid

All of us are on a unique journey. No two stories are the same. Chances are, if you picked up this book, you and I share some common threads in our tapestries.

Burnout is a disease nobody talks about until it's too late. Statistics and stories prove that the health of those serving in ministry is declining — spiritually, physically, emotionally, and relationally.

At some point along the road, your heart, your mind, your spirit —maybe even your body — have been damaged while fighting the battles of good and evil.

Mine too.

When we should have been fighting with our fellow believers back-to-back, we find ourselves bandaging our wounds from friendly fire.

When we should be breathing life into a comatose world, we find ourselves gasping for air, just trying to survive.

When we should be celebrating the gift of our friends and families, we find our hearts breaking for the way they are mistreated.

A very real pain comes out of a very real battle each of us is called to fight. To some of us, this is a relatively new and maybe even a surprising pain. To others, we've grown numb because we've learned to expect the worse and feeling nothing is better than feeling the pain we think is just around the corner.

You may be taking your first steps into serving God. Or maybe like me, you've been exposed to both the beautiful and terrible faces of the church for your entire life.

Although our stories may be different, we are unified in at least one very clear and very special way: It is obvious that God has placed a burden on your heart to see the church, and the world, healed and restored.

Me too.

So I wanted to share a little bit of my own background, with the intent that you'll not only get to know the woman behind the words but also relate to some part of my life — whether my childhood, my time away from the church, my own season of burnout or even that exciting feeling of the Spirit stirring in your heart when you've come to rest in Him, whole and healed.

Hi. I'm Anne, and I Was Born in a Church (Kind of, Anyway)

Even before my dad was a pastor, we spent almost every waking moment at church. My mom was in the choir, my dad taught various classes, and I hung out in the nursery with the other toddlers.

When I was five, my father took a pastoral position at a small church in Circle Back, Texas. It was his first full-time position out of seminary, and he got paid a stately $200 per week. My mother stayed at home and took care of my baby brother. On weekends, my dad and I would go fishing and rock hunting.

Everything seemed normal. We were a happy, small town, pastor's family.

At least for a little while.

A few years later, we moved to a farming community in west Texas. Although my father's paycheck was only slightly more, his time away from our family had exponentially increased. He'd come home later and later at night. He was tired. Although we'd still go fishing, our plans seemed to be interrupted more often than not.

Once a month, he'd have a deacons meeting. I began noticing that when he came home from these particular meetings, he'd be upset. He'd make sure my brother and I were in bed before he and my mom would have closed-door discussions.

Some might call it being nosy, but I like to call it being curious. Even after using the "glass to the wall" trick I had seen on television, I could never make out specific words of my parents' conversations…but the tone was unmistakable.

Something was terribly wrong, and I needed to know what it was.

With my mom starting to teach to supplement our income and my dad always being gone, I was responsible for taking care of my younger brother. I'd give him some Ninja Turtles to keep him occupied, and I'd begin to pore over my Nancy Drew books.

Why?

I had a mystery to solve. And I needed to learn how to spy.

I began setting up an infallible plan to listen in on the next deacons meeting.

Deacons Meeting Espionage

The deacons meetings always took place in the fellowship hall, and much to my benefit, there was a janitor's closet adjacent to the room. I had another thing working for me. There was an exterior door that opened into the janitor's closet.

Over the next week, I snuck into the church and began building a small fort of tables in the corner of the janitor's closet. I angled the tables so that when I entered the closet through the exterior door, I'd be completely hidden.

The Sunday of the deacons meeting approached. During the morning service, I left the auditorium to use the bathroom, making another stop along the way. I put my spy kit — a Trapper Keeper folder with a photo of two kittens on it, my favorite four-colored pen, and a small tape recorder — underneath the tables. I also unlocked the exterior door, ensuring I'd be able to easily enter the room later that evening.

I could barely contain my excitement that day, anticipating my mission that night. I went home after the service and told my mom I was going to bed early. She eventually went outside to the utility room to do laundry.

That's when I made my escape.

I swiftly traveled from our parsonage to the church next door and quietly entered through the exterior door to the janitor's closet.

My plan was perfect.

The meeting had just started, and I could hear everyone's voice clearly. I pressed the play+record combination on the tape recorder, just to make sure I didn't miss anything.

One of the four deacons said an opening prayer. Another began the meeting by summarizing the previous month's attendance and finances and giving updates on hospitalized members who had been visited.

Boring . . .

I began doodling on my paper until I heard my dad mention the word vacation.

"Well, the kids are heading back to school next month, and since my father's cancer is spreading, I thought I'd take my yearly vacation in a few weeks to have the family visit my parents in Fort Worth."

Sweet! I love staying with my grandparents! Please say yes, please say yes, please say yes.

The room was unexpectedly quiet. I heard a metal folding chair squeak, and a deacon, who was also the music director, said in his angry, thick Texas accent, "Brother Ron, now, you know you already took your vacation back in May when you went to Russia. You can't expect for us to be alright with you takin' another one."

My dad paused, and then replied, "The trip to Russia? Brother Chuck, that was an association mission trip. You know that. My family didn't go."

Brother Chuck didn't seem too impressed. He growled, "Still sounds like a vacation to me!"

One thing I've always loved about my dad is the deliberately slow and patient tone with which he speaks. Even in the most ridiculous situations, he manages to keep an almost frighteningly calm demeanor.

"If you consider visiting a Communist nation and being followed by the KGB as you try to discreetly hand out Bibles a vacation, I suppose you're correct."

Oh. So that's where I get my passive-aggressive sarcasm.

I could hear the other deacons begin to grumble. The lead deacon who moderated the meeting interrupted the next livid remark Brother Chuck was beginning to make. "Chuck, you know very well it was a church-sponsored and approved mission trip. Brother Ron, I hope you and your family have a great time visiting your folks. Let's move on."

My fourth grade brain couldn't comprehend what happened. I knew adults disagreed, but this was our music leader. I had never heard him speak so harshly, and I didn't understand why only one of the deacons had defended my father. I thought these people were his friends!

I didn't have much time to dwell on these thoughts before Chuck started talking again. This time, however, his words came from left field.

"You know, Brother Ron. You are a liar."

EXCUSE ME? I almost flew out of the janitor's closet and punched sweet Brother Chuck in his face. My heart pounded, and I desperately wanted to defend my dad.

I took a deep breath and managed to stay put.

A good spy never lets emotions get in the way of the mission.

My dad, seemingly unfazed by this remark, asked what would lead Chuck to make such a terrible accusation.

Chuck replied, "I saw you park your cars on the church parking lot instead of on your driveway this weekend. You're trying to make it look like we've got more people here — and we can't have a liar for a pastor. So I'm going to ask you to resign at the next business meeting."

My dad reminded Chuck of the landscaping being done at the parsonage and that the cars had to be moved out of our driveway until it was taken care of. The church had approved the expense and the work a few months ago.

Chuck mumbled something about how he must have missed that meeting.

After dealing with a few other minor issues, the group began a time of prayer to close out the meeting. I closed up shop and left. Checking to make sure my mom was in my parents' bedroom as I predicted her to be, I came through the house's side door and managed to get into my bedroom undetected.

A few minutes later, my dad came home, exhausted. I heard him ask if we were in bed as he closed the door to their room. Through the walls I could hear my mom cry as Dad shared the meeting's "highlights."

I didn't sleep much that night. My heart was still racing, and my stomach felt a little sick from hearing people who were supposedly closest to my dad tear him apart and refuse to come to his defense. These were Christian men. I went to school with their children. We would eat at their homes, and they'd come over to ours.

A little bit of my world crashed in on me that night.

And I wish I would have known that this night was only the beginning.

A Fiery Escaping to a Fire Escape

Needless to say, things only got worse at that church. My father eventually resigned and took another pastoring position in a town two hours away.

I was thirteen and had fallen back into the role of the good preacher's kid. The church seemed healthy, my dad was home more, and I assumed we'd be there for a very long time. I remember my dad saying he thought he could retire from this church.

Three years later, another hopeful circumstance turned ugly.

One night, my dad received a phone call from Stanley, one of his closest friends and mentors, who also happened to be a deacon. He told my father that an impromptu leaders meeting had been called earlier that day — and my dad had intentionally not been invited. Stanley had gone to the meeting because he knew that the man who organized it had a tendency to stir up trouble in the church, and he wanted to be there to bring some balance.

The issue was evangelism — kind of. My father is very passionate about evangelism and outreach to the community. He had planned several classes for members to learn why and how somebody shares Christ. Over three quarters of the people in the town we were living in didn't go to church — so the stakes for life change were huge!

However, a younger group of leaders in the church believed that because my dad was being paid to do ministry, his attempts to get the entire church involved in outreach was only "slacking off." They made similar accusations toward our part-time youth pastor.

My dad realized that his options were limited.

A few months later, at a regularly scheduled business meeting, my dad read a letter to the church announcing his "forced" resignation.

He said nobody was holding a gun to his head (I mean, this was Texas), but his love for unity was forcing him to step down. He told the members about the issues that, if not dealt with, would cause a split, and because he cared more for their health as a body, he was going to step away from this ministry.

A few members asked questions and told my father he didn't need to leave. Most of the church sat quietly, with deer-in-the-headlights looks on their faces. The core group of antagonists began to make absurd threats about what they'd do to my family if my dad didn't step down. A few stood up and defended his outreach plans.

It became a very messy meeting.

The feeling of frustration I had experienced several years before quickly returned, and it was now coupled with teenage angst and courage. Armed with years of Awana and Bible drills, I quickly flipped to Ephesians 4:3, stood up, interrupted what was going on, cleared my throat loudly, and read, "Make every effort to keep the unity of the Spirit through the bond of peace."

I continued in a shaky voice. "How can you even call yourselves Christians when all you do is fight? This is just . . . stupid!"

I was met with a mixture of apathy and silence. I closed my Bible, picked up the notebook I always kept with me, and stormed out, slamming the large wooden door behind me. As quickly as I could, I ran over to our education building and climbed the fire escape. Under the glow and buzz of a nearby streetlight, I furiously wrote a letter to God in my journal with the small, golf scorecard pencil I had gotten out of the back of a pew.

I gave God a choice that night (sixteen-year-olds are so smart!). Either I was going to part ways with the church entirely, or he was going to give me a way to help bring unity to the church.

I'll admit that it was a big prayer for a sixteen-year-old. And I'm not quite sure how I knew what it all meant. I just knew that my heart had been set on fire — and if God would let me, my sole purpose in life had just been defined.

So I waited.

Silence

I didn't receive an answer that night, or anytime shortly thereafter, so I assumed God didn't care. After my father resigned, my family moved to Dallas so we could be closer to my aging grandparents and so my mom could take a teaching job.

Several months after moving, my dad still hadn't found employment. He would occasionally look for jobs, but because he was so burned out from ministry, none of the ones he applied for were in a church. And I'm sure that many of you know that finding a job in the marketplace is nearly impossible after having difficulty defining your role in a church. He was clearly depressed. My dad spent most of his time in my parents' bedroom. The spark in his eyes was gone.

Going to church was a very rare occurrence. The heaviness in our house was palpable.

How could the church do this? How could God let this happen?

Seeing the state of my family — both financially and emotionally — broke my heart even more. When I was seventeen, I decided to graduate from high school a year early and move out. I didn't want to be a burden financially. I turned down a few scholarships to some colleges I applied for, decided not to go to school right away, and instead worked full time managing a Christian bookstore.

But that was all a front. I was an empty shell, thinking my good-girl exterior would compensate for my dying heart. In the shadows of my life, I was medicating years of hurt by escaping. I was compulsively looking at pornography, which led to having inappropriate relationships, and I even began combining alcohol with prescription anxiety medicine — all to numb the pain I was feeling from my past experiences with church and other failed relationships.

After seeing even more brokenness in my job with the "Christian" bookstore, I decided I was through with anything Jesus. I got a job working at a trendy Dallas dot-com. The new job only fueled my need and my ability to find resources for medicating my hurt. I couldn't bear the pain of my past — or the person I was allowing myself to become.

Hints of a Savior

In the middle of this downward spiral, Lexie, my best friend from high school, and I unexpectedly reconnected. Lexie decided that she needed to take a break from college, and she moved into my Dallas condo.

The very first Sunday after she had moved in, she woke me up at the crack of dawn and asked me where I went to church.

I covered my head up with my duvet and mumbled incoherently.

She decided to find a church on her own. By the time she came back, I was barely pulling myself out of bed.

"You're coming with me next week, OK?"

God definitely had Lexie there for a reason. She slowly began to infuse our relationship with a Christlike love and grace. Although she let me know she couldn't stand to watch me do all the things I was doing, she was always there to make sure I was OK.

Through a mutual friend, we met a youth pastor who worked at a church a couple of hours away on the Texas/Oklahoma border. Even though it was a bit of a drive, Lexie and I began attending his church every other Sunday. The youth pastor took a genuine interest in some of the issues I had been facing.

I felt I could trust him, so I opened up. He emailed me certain Scriptures he was praying for me, and I felt my heart beginning to soften. I quit drinking as much and stopped hanging out with some of the people who weren't the best influence in my life. I left my job at the dot-com and took a much more focused position at a design agency.

For the first time in a long time, I began giving in to the gentle songs God had begun to sing to my heart.

Toto, We're in Kansas

Lexie and I continued attending the church in Oklahoma, and even though their charismatic methodology was much different from my traditional Baptist upbringing, God was clearly moving, and the small taste of what I experienced gave me the slightest bit of hope.

Five months after Lexie moved to Dallas, I found out that my department at work was being downsized and my job was going to be eliminated within a few short weeks.

I talked to Lexie about the situation, and she suggested we move to Kansas for a fresh start.

The Midwest seemed safe and cheap enough. We had some friends in the Kansas City area. A week after my last day at the agency, we packed everything in a friend's van and my little sports car and headed up to the Sunflower State.

Since we were new, it was easy to blow off the church thing again. I had to find a job and become acquainted with the new city, right?

Several months after we had moved, some friends of ours who were in a band were playing at a church near our new apartment. We decided to go and hear them play.

The moment I stepped into the church, my heart raced and my stomach tightened up into an uncomfortable little ball. I couldn't breathe. I started to sweat.

Lexie went up near the stage, but I stayed in the back of the auditorium. I sat hidden in a corner and tried to figure out what was happening. Was I sick? Was I having a panic attack? Maybe I had just had too much coffee.

It's Not the Coffee

Remember the ultimatum I gave God on the fire escape?

Almost five years later, I got my answer.

I want you here. This is my church. This is my bride. Remember your father? Remember your pain? This is my church. This is my bride. I want you here. I will give you what you need. I will open up doors. And now is your time, if you'll let me. I want you here.

At the age of twenty-one, I was officially freaked out. And evidently, I was wearing my feelings on my sleeve.

A spunky redheaded girl around my age came up to me. She stuck out her hand. I shook it, still in shock from what I had just heard.

"Hi, I'm Kristi."

I think I told her my name.

"So can I pray with you?"

I stared up at her, dazed, and must have nodded my head yes.

She pulled me behind a partition and prayed for me. She prayed for me to have friends. And then she prayed for my involvement with the church – that church, specifically.

What? My heart began pounding even harder. Why would she say that?

Kristi said amen and then asked the big question.

"So I work at this church, and I really think you'd make a great table leader for our youth group. Interested?"

I politely declined.

Coming up with reasons to avoid church was completely second nature to me. I told her I hadn't been to church much in the last few years and was probably not the best example for students. I was really busy with my new job and would hate to over commit.

She smiled, said she understood, and then asked if I'd mind having coffee with her sometime. We exchanged numbers, and within a few weeks we were hanging out pretty regularly.

After a little while, Kristi twisted my arm, and I agreed to help her out for one night at the church.

That one night turned into a year of volunteering.

And that year of volunteering turned into a full-time job offer in the student ministry where I had been serving.

Once again, I declined the offer. I wanted to focus on my career and on my transitioning to the Midwest. My preference was to continue serving as a volunteer.

But I left out one very important reason.

I had promised myself that I would never, ever, EVER work in a church.

Never Say Never

A couple of months after turning down the job, I was hit with a virus that kept me in bed for almost two straight weeks. With nothing to do but lie flat on my back, I felt this unrelenting impression that I needed to call Chad, our student pastor, and talk to him about the job.

I picked up my phone, dialed, and hung up.

I just couldn't do it. I was terrified to work at a church.

I could not take a chance and be hurt again. So deeply, deeply hurt.

As I reached to put my phone back on my night table, it rang.

It was Chad.

We talked about the position — about some of my reservations, but mostly about how, over the last two weeks, both of us were completely positive I was supposed to accept this role in ministry.

Even though I was so scared that I could have thrown up all over the place, I accepted the job.

I said yes.

I knew my life would never be the same.

Chapter 2: Comparing Cows and Churches

In front of me sat a large pile of cattle carcasses, still smoldering from the fire that had destroyed them. Occasionally, I'd hear a crackle or pop coming from the heap, but for the most part, the grassy English field was silent.

Thankfully, I was four thousand miles away, cozied up in my apartment and watching this on TV, far removed from the smells that would have been carried by the damp winds. I was tuned in to a BBC channel, viewing a documentary about bovine spongiform encephalopathy, an affliction better known as mad cow disease.

Now, mad cow disease is a pretty odd ailment that, in most cases, only infects cows. And, as I would learn in the documentary, it has four unique characteristics:

1. The disease lies dormant for a given amount of time, going unnoticed. It can be a period of months to a few years before the disease is found.

2. Mad cow disease is caused by a mutated protein that attaches itself to the cow's central nervous system, thus affecting the cow's brain and responses (hence the name). Essentially, it turns the cow's brain and spinal cord into a spongy-type matter. Slowly, the cow's mental and physical health begins to deteriorate.

3. Mad cow disease is transmitted by cows eating the suspect protein. Since cows are often fed the remains of other cattle (something called meat and bone meal), it's easy for an entire herd to become infected at once if they share the same food source.

4. Mad cow disease ultimately leads to the infected cow's death. There is no cure.

In the United Kingdom, the disease had reached epidemic proportions. Because of its ability to spread to both cattle and humans, over four million cattle were killed as a precaution.

Now, if humans were to contract mad cow disease through infected meat, they would share the same fate as the cows. Neurological functions would begin to slow down, causing psychosis, uncontrollable body movements, and eventually coma and death.

What struck me about mad cow disease was its similarity to the phenomenon of burnout in the church. (Don't ask me how my brain made that leap. All I know is that it did, and here we are!) We'll explore the similarities below.

What You Can't See Can Hurt You

The first characteristic, the fact that the disease is unnoticed for a period of time, couldn't be truer in the context of burnout.

Remember the job I accepted in student ministry?

The church was in a rapidly growing community, and my new job couldn't have been better. Our team chemistry was nothing short of amazing. The momentum grew, the number of kids whose lives were changed grew, our staff grew — and everything was healthy and thriving. Soon our one weekly service became two, and we started planning our own camps and mission trips.

Things were going so well. We were on top of the world. It seemed too good to be true.

And it was.

Because I loved my job so much, I (proudly) didn't take a single vacation day during my first year on staff. By the end of our summer camp (which I was responsible to manage), I was exhausted.

Needless to say, the quickness of the onset of my weariness caught me off guard. The job I had once looked forward to tackling every single workday (and sometimes on my days off) I was now dreading.

Since I had allowed spending time with God to be replaced by spending time doing things for God, my spiritual tank had been sucked dry. When that happened, I began to lose perspective on almost every area of my life. My defenses were down, and I allowed myself to start believing the little lies the enemy would throw into my path.

> *You know, they are totally taking advantage of you. With your experience in management, they should be paying you double what you're making.*
>
> *Do you really think what you're doing matters? You're just a little girl on the support staff. Nobody really cares what you think. You'll never be able to lead like one of the guys. It's just the world you're in.*
>
> *And all that stuff you see and hear in staff meetings? You know this place is nothing but egos and trouble.*
>
> *Come on. You know you shouldn't be working in this church world. You shouldn't even be in a church. Life was so much better when you could pretend these things didn't exist.*

The smart thing at this point would have been to talk to somebody about what I was going through, but ministry was supposed to be so professional — so perfect.

I kept quiet.

As these thoughts were allowed to simmer silently over the course of a few weeks, I became more convinced these voices were right, so I started looking for a job back in the marketplace. Back where it didn't matter what your gender or your age was. If you put in the time, had the ideas, and made it to happy hour, you'd have all the respect you need to make it to the top.

However, when my efforts proved fruitless, I was discouraged. I actually began feeling guilty about working at the church, since there were so many people who would kill for the chance to be in vocational ministry.

Then out of left field, our church's administrator and senior pastor approached me about a new position that had been created —director of communication and media.

Director? The word seemed to shimmer and glimmer with prestige and power.

This new position would allow me to use my marketing and communications background. I'd oversee all areas of communication and media for the weekend services. I'd get to manage two creative teams. I'd get my own office. I'd be the youngest person on our leadership staff.

Director. Director. *Director*! That sure had a nice ring to it!

I was in. This had to be the answer! I told our youth pastor I was going to be changing positions. He asked me to reconsider and told me I was probably letting the exhaustion of our intense summer schedule get the best of me. Deep down, I think I knew he was right, but I was dead set on taking the new position (and the new salary, the new office, etcetera). So after helping with the transition of bringing in a new hire to our student staff, I moved over to the administration offices, high and lofty, on the second floor of a bank building. I'd be rubbing elbows with our senior leadership staff every day.

This was it! This was the good life.

Like most new things, every aspect of my new position was perfect. My strengths in problem solving and management were being put to good use, as both the communication and media areas were a mess. I was asked to help brand the church, redo the website, strengthen our weekend experiences, and involve and equip new volunteers.

I thought things were intense in student ministry, but the new position made my old schedule look like a summer vacation. Because our church was bursting at the seams, we had services on Saturday nights and all day on Sundays. We also had an off-site venue with multiple service times. My scheduled day off was Friday, but I'd often find myself finalizing weekend logistics on Friday afternoon and evening.

It was the only way to get it done. And, hey — it was all "for God." I believed thousands of people were relying on my talent every weekend to help engage them in their worship experience. Everything had to be perfect. I would settle for nothing less.

And as time went by, I was still none the wiser to the fact that my pride and I were continuing on a downward spiral.

A close friend and I talked about my schedule constantly, and I'd always promise to do a better job of taking time off. But I never kept those promises. He warned me if I kept burning the candle at both ends, I would eventually burn out.

I refused to believe him.

And he was right.

About six months into my new position, I started feeling some tightness in my chest and had difficulty breathing. My doctor sent me to an allergy and asthma doctor, who in turn discovered I had pretty severe acid reflux. He scheduled an esophagogastroduodenoscopy (also known as an EGD), which is pretty much a fancy way of saying, "You get to swallow a camera so we can make sure your esophagus hasn't disintegrated."

The test was over quickly and found nothing too remarkable —just some minor inflammation that could easily be healed. They told me that if I experienced any stomach pain or peculiar symptoms for the next day or so, I should come back, as there was a slight risk they could have punctured my stomach during the procedure.

Hmmm. That's nice to know.

Expecting nothing out of the ordinary, I hung out at home on my day off. Somewhere around noon, I went from very normal to very sick — very quickly.

I drove myself back to the hospital where they had performed the procedure. They quickly admitted me to the ER and did some blood work and a CT scan.

"We think you might have appendicitis, but we're not sure. The CT showed you have abdominal inflammation, but your blood work is fine. To be safe, we're going to admit you, start you on some antibiotics, and watch you for a while."

Appendicitis isn't the end of the world. I was a little freaked out about the possibility of having surgery (and probably more freaked out that I'd have to miss work unexpectedly), but I was relieved I wasn't bleeding internally. They gave me some medicine for my pain and scheduled some tests for the next day.

One day of tests led to two. Two quickly became five. Each day it seemed my pain increased. And after every test, the doctor would come in and say the same thing.

"Well, we still haven't found a cause for your inflammation and pain. So tomorrow, we're going to do more tests."

I thought I'd never get out of the hospital. Or eat again. I felt like I was on an episode of House.

After a week, and after what seemed like every test they could run had been performed, a couple of the doctors came in with some theories as to my ailment. One of them asked how my stress level was.

I explained my schedule and the demands of my position at the church, justifying it with the fact I was only twenty-five and really in perfect health. A little stress never killed anyone.

And then one of the doctors explained to me that if I didn't change my lifestyle, I'd probably be back in the hospital within the year.

Unhealthy from All Angles

Another interesting element to mad cow disease is the way in which it affects all areas of the cow's health. The cows begin suffering both physical and mental symptoms. They begin to lose their ability in muscle coordination, and in the most advanced stages they deteriorate socially, isolating themselves from their herd. Cows begin to display abnormal behaviors, including aggression and fear.

Unlike our bovine friends, we have an additional area that makes up our health. We share the physical, mental, and social (what I'll call relational) aspects with the cows, but we also have spiritual health to take into consideration. Even though these areas do affect us in their own unique ways, they also overlap into each other (see illustration).

At the time, it was obvious that my physical health was suffering. As I lay for days in a hospital bed, cocktails of medicines being injected into my bloodstream, I couldn't help but wonder what damage my decisions had caused in other areas. Obviously the damage that had accumulated over the last three years had also affected my heart — one thing God wants completely.

After my trip to the hospital, my body was undergoing healing, but the other areas of my health continued to decline. Even though I was becoming stronger physically, the deepest sense of who I was had wilted away so slowly, I didn't even realize it.

My emotional health probably suffered the most noticeable damage. I sometimes dealt with long bouts of excessive worry before, but during this period, worry consumed me. I was anxious about my health, anxious because I knew I was dropping the ball, anxious that someone would break into my house, anxious to drive, anxious that I would have a meltdown — and that's just the start!

Because of all the worry, I began losing sleep (which only made matters worse). Relationally, I began withdrawing from friendships and accountability because I didn't want anyone to think I was weak for struggling with so many things. I always needed to be the strong one. The dependable one. The rock. It was the only way I thought I could make it in ministry.

The lack of personal interaction, along with my fear and lack of sleep, put me into a depression. Even getting out of bed was a chore, and some days I didn't make it.

My relationship with God during this time was desperate but unfocused. Still believing the lie that I could save the world by myself, I didn't know what to pray for. I felt like a failure as a Christ-follower because I couldn't keep my act together enough to make a difference in the world — which was the cry of my heart.

One of our associate pastors — a good friend — noticed the confusion I was wearing on my sleeve once I returned to the office after my hospital stay. He came into my office, and we talked about the things I had experienced.

As important as my physical wake-up call was, it was nothing compared to the impact of the question he asked me: "Does working at this church interfere with your communion with Christ?"

Huh? Are you asking me if serving is hurting my relationship with God? Isn't that a paradox? How could that be possible?

I sat in my chair, stunned. With nothing left to do but say what both of us were thinking, I replied, "Yes."

But how could it? How could working in a church with an amazing staff, serving a wonderful community, all for God, interfere with my own relationship with my Father?

I didn't have the answer. But I knew, beyond a shadow of a doubt, that I was so wrapped up in doing, I had forgotten how to simply be.

How to be a child to a Father

How to be a vessel he can use

How to be a light in a dark world

My friend's question haunted me for weeks.

Contamination

I always thought cows ate grass. Evidently, this isn't always the case. In Europe, where mad cow disease was first discovered, cows were being fed a sheep by-product meal mixed with their grain. The meal contained a mutated sheep protein called prion, which, when ingested, changes into a harmful agent and infects the cow with the disease. In the 1990s, when the outbreak of mad cow disease spread throughout the United Kingdom, it was the result of the cattle industry beginning to feed rendered, prion-infected bovine meat and bone meal to young calves.[1]

It's pretty gross, but cows became infected with the disease by eating the by-products of other infected cattle.

In both positions I had at the church, I know that my unhealthy attitude affected those around me. I worked closely with other staff and dozens of volunteers and projected my high expectations on them. If I gave up my nights and weekends, I assumed they would do the same. There was almost an unhealthy competitiveness in my spirit. If my boss came in early, I had to be there earlier. If she stayed late, I'd wait until after she'd leave to go home.

Oh, and I wanted to prove that I loved Jesus more.

At least, that was what I believed.

I thought the more I sacrificed, the more I loved Jesus. The more hours I put in for God's work, the more I was committed to his cause. I wanted to make my God proud, and I did a great job at it.

The only problem? God wasn't my God. My pride was my god.

Sometimes our environments contribute to the expectations we have as volunteers, as family members, or as church staff members.

The fear of letting people down, especially in spiritual matters, can often cause us to feel obligated or pressured into meeting unrealistic expectations, or worse, spending more time doing things for God instead of being what God wants us to be. That can lead to serious stress.

What's worse, it's easy for the resulting attitudes to contaminate a team or even an entire church.

Nothing will inhibit the Spirit from working in the church (as in all of us, not just your church) faster than bitterness. Than anger. Than pride. Than envy. Than laziness. Than lust. Than gossip. All of these things are deeply rooted issues that can spread and contaminate an entire body.

We become sick. When we're sick, how can we show a dying world health? When we're hopeless, how can we show hope? We can't.

Someone's Out to Destroy You

I can imagine Satan hanging out in a recliner with his feet propped up, thinking what a fantastic job he did stealing, killing, and destroying me during that very hard season in my life. Slowly and subtly, my defenses weakened and I allowed myself to be taken down. And not only did he take me down; the decisions I made affected my coworkers, my friends, and my church family.

Mad church disease can and will strip away everything from your identity — from who you are in Christ. Why? Because the chief bearer of the disease only wants to destroy you.

John in his gospel records what Jesus said to a crowd of listeners:

"The thief comes only to steal and kill and destroy" (John 10:10a).

I realize this is a verse you are probably very familiar with — but that fact doesn't make it any less true. And I'd like to point out one word: "The thief comes only to steal and kill and destroy" (emphasis mine).

Only.

> Only.

>> ONLY!

The one objective the enemy has is to steal, kill, and destroy you. You may have heard somebody say, "If you're doing really good work for the Lord, Satan's going to try to stop you," or, "When you're really a threat to the devil, that's when he'll attack the hardest."

I don't think there is an "if" or a "when" about it. Satan is out to destroy you no matter what!

And if Satan can put things in your path to trip you up and take others down with you, I'm sure there's no better way he'd rather spend his time. He's going to ask himself how he can kill as many birds with one stone as possible. When the death and destruction of Christ-followers is the main goal, the enemy is going to think strategically.

Cows don't have much hope when they are infected with mad cow disease. Even though the process can take years, they die. There's no vaccine. We're a bit more fortunate. Satan's sole purpose in life is to ruin us — but God's sole purpose in life is to redeem us.

Cows don't get a second chance — but we are promised a second chance, and more.

The rest of Jesus' statement in John 10:10 reads,

"I have come that they may have life, and have it to the full."

And that's the amazing thing about grace. Regardless of how we struggle or how we fall, regardless of how many people are affected by our actions, God is a God of healing. God is a God of restoration and life.

Satan loves to steal and destroy what God has intended for good. He wants us to kill our ministry, our passion, and our hope so that we're useless. Through Christ, we're made complete. It's time to truly realize that — and begin to claim back what is rightfully ours.

Second Opinion

Bill Hybels, senior pastor,

Willow Creek Community Church, South Barrington, Illinois

A. M. M.: You've mentioned that you've come close to being sidelined from ministry a couple of times. What led you to that place, and how did you recognize that what you were experiencing was endangering what you refer to as your "holy discontent"?

B. H.: On two occasions I allowed the growth of our church and the growth of the international component of what we do to lead to a level of stress that became unhealthy. It didn't quench my passion for the local church; I just realized that I was going to have to pace myself differently, organize the staff and my colleagues for more effective service, and change internal structures and procedures so that I could continue to pursue my God-given passions in a healthy way as opposed to getting overly exhausted or psychologically worn down.

A. M. M.: What boundaries did you set up in your life, both personally and professionally, that helped to keep you from moving into a self-reliant mode?

B. H.: I'm a firm believer in the spiritual disciplines. For example, I'm very committed to a pattern of solitude — secret acts of service, prayer, and journaling. I try to engage in daily journaling to chronicle the activity of God in my life and to help me sort out the complexities and the distractions that always seem to crop up. I'm also quite disciplined with my workday. I leave the office between 4:00 and 4:30 almost every single day. I watch how many nights in a row I'm out in a given ministry week. I take Sunday afternoons and Mondays off every single week, and in the summertime, I take a summer study break to allow a physical and emotional and spiritual "refilling" of sorts to counterbalance the "output" mode that typically characterizes my life.

A. M. M.: Once someone identifies his or her "holy discontent" — such as serving the poor or eradicating treatable diseases or helping people repair tenuous marriages or enfolding wounded people into community — it's easy for them to care so much about that particular firestorm-of-frustration issue that they unintentionally fall into a pattern of obsessive thoughts and behaviors in their noble attempt to join God in his kingdom-building activity. Sometimes exhaustion even sets in. What advice do you have for church leaders and their families for pursuing their areas of holy discontent in God-honoring ways?

B. H.: I like to look at that whole subject matter holistically. To engage in a cycle of working incredibly hard and then resting up is to rejuvenate only partially. There must also be consideration given to what you're reading, who you're surrounding yourself with, and what recreational activities you're pursuing that will genuinely refill your tanks. Especially as leaders in the church, we consistently need to be filled up and buoyed in our spirits because everybody takes their cue from the leader. If the leader is exhausted, then the people following that leader will feel exhausted. If the leader is wearing thin on hope, then people start losing hope too. If the leader gets pessimistic, everybody gets pessimistic. You see where this is going.

A. M. M.: What are some of the diseases you see plaguing the church today?

B. H.: I see twin towers of concern. One is burnout; the other is complacency. There are a lot of Christ-followers who haven't taken the time to figure out what their holy discontent is, and so they're doing a gradual slide into apathy and complacency — and that is unconscionable in a broken and lost world. I'm as concerned about Christ-followers' apathy as I am about other believers who are borderline exhausted. I would hope we could find the kind of energy that comes only from the Holy Spirit so that we can sustain productive, Christ-honoring ministry over the long haul.

Chapter 3: The Emergency

When the notion of writing this book first struck me, I did a little bit of research. A couple of things surprised me.

First, there aren't very many books or readily available resources dealing with burnout in ministry. An online book search gave me a handful of results when I looked for the words "Church" and "Burnout" in titles. Out of that small number, only a couple of the books were still in print. That led me to wonder if there was even a need for discussion of this topic. Maybe the lack of books and resources meant a lack of interest.

I decided to probe a bit further and created an anonymous, online questionnaire to see what people were thinking about burnout —if they were thinking anything at all. Since I knew that burnout didn't just affect people on church staffs but families and volunteers/members as well, questions were developed for all three groups.

In July 2007, a website was launched, and with the help of a viral social media campaign, within just a couple of days almost a thousand people had taken the surveys. My email account was actually shut down by my provider due to the increased number of emails I was receiving and sending. They thought I was a spammer! Multitudes of people were sharing their stories, their struggles with working in ministry, and their feelings about it all — feelings they thought they could never share with anyone.

And the second thing that surprised me? A resounding voice was crying out, "I am burned-out! And evidently I'm not alone. I thought I was the only one."

Now these surveys weren't scientific in any way, but they did capture a snapshot of what a number of people involved in ministry were experiencing and provide some noteworthy demographics.

Noteworthy Questionnaire Results

Location: As we looked at the responses, the locations of people who responded to the questionnaires proved interesting. Although most were from the United States, people from every continent but Antarctica participated. There were pastors from Peru, volunteers from New Zealand, wives of pastors from Scotland, staff leaders in Malaysia and Egypt and Turkey and Hong Kong. And that's just the tip of the iceberg.

Age: Another interesting finding was the ages of people who answered questions. We were assuming that a majority of responses would come from Gen X and Gen Y, yet surprisingly many people in their fifties — even sixties and seventies — completed the questionnaire.

Position in leadership: The people who were interested in the concept of mad church disease weren't just pastors. Besides spouses, children, or siblings of those in ministry, practically any position you could dream up in a church was represented. Pastors of all kinds, from lead pastors to worship pastors to children's pastors — as well as those holding a variety of support staff roles and creative roles, even those with the all-encompassing title of "worker bee" — showed they had experienced burnout or knew of someone who had.

Length of time in ministry: Another non-discriminating factor for ministry burnout is the length of time spent in ministry. From just a few weeks in ministry to almost forty years, the ministry span of those affected by mad church disease is vast.

Accountability: Most people who responded to the survey had some kind of accountability in place, such as an accountability partner. Many people desire to have that person in their life; however, most people indicated they had, at some point in time, not been honest with that person.

Tangible effects: Almost every person who completed the questionnaire said the stress from ministry had affected them either emotionally (most common were feelings of worthlessness, depression, anxiety, anger, or loneliness) or physically (most common problems were insomnia, headaches, stomach problems, heart issues, weight gain, or inflammation).

Bible study: When asked about spending time in Bible study, apart from "studying for sermons or teaching," a quarter of those who responded said they didn't.

Moving On to Scientific Research

Realizing that my online questionnaire wasn't scientific and was a bit biased, I continued researching to see if there was any scientific data that would confirm the prevalence of burnout symptoms in the church.

Ellison Research, a research firm located in Phoenix, Arizona, has conducted several studies of the health of ministers and ministers' families.[1] These studies, conducted from 2002 to 2005 in all fifty states of the United States, spanned all Protestant denominations and sizes. I was excited to see if their scientific research would confirm my own findings and feelings.

Physical Health

When I started vocational ministry in 2003, I was right around my ideal weight for my height. I also started working in ministry that year. Now, I'm not saying that the two are entirely related, or that ministry "made" me gain weight, but because I didn't manage my schedule and plan my meals well, over the course of the next three to four years, I gained thirty to forty pounds! Realizing the damage this was causing me, I took steps to lose the weight I gained. I'm now back down to a healthy weight, but I know if I'm not careful, I could quickly pack on the pounds and harm my body by what I consume.

Insomnia and other sleep issues are also prevalent in the culture and within the church. According to a 2003 study, sleep deprivation costs $150 billion each year in higher stress and reduced worker productivity.[2]

Physical health is not a topic the Bible shies away from. David in Psalm 139 writes of our bodies as being fearfully and wonderfully created by God. I like the cut-and-dried approach Paul takes in 1 Corinthians 6:20: "You were bought at a price. Therefore honor God with your body."

It's easy to neglect our physical health when we're faced with the demands of ministry — whether it's our vocation or whether we've chosen to volunteer. Unfortunately, many of us take our health for granted.

The 568 senior pastors surveyed by Ellison Research were described as "not in terribly good shape physically." Collectively, they averaged less than seven hours of sleep per night, were more than thirty pounds overweight, and maintained poor eating habits.[3]

Eating Habits/Weight Issues

- 71 percent of all ministers admitted to being overweight by an average of 32.1 pounds. One-third of all ministers were overweight by at least 25 pounds, including 15 percent who were overweight by 50 pounds or more.

- Two-thirds of all pastors skip a meal at least one day a week, and 39 percent skip meals three or more days a week.

- 83 percent eat food once a week that they know they shouldn't because it is unhealthy, including 41 percent who do this three or more days a week.

- 88 percent eat fast food at least one day a week, and 33 percent eat fast food three or more days a week.

- 50 percent get the recommended minimum amount of exercise (30 minutes per day, three times a week); 28 percent don't exercise at all.

Stress-related Health Issues

- Four out of ten ministers (approximately 39 percent) reported digestive problems once a week, with 14 percent having chronic digestive problems (three days per week).

- 87 percent don't get enough sleep at least once a week, with almost half (47 percent) getting less sleep than they need at least three nights a week. Only 16 percent regularly get the recommendation of eight hours or more per night.
- 52 percent experience physical symptoms of stress at least once a week, and nearly one out of four experiences physical symptoms three or more times a week.

Ron Sellers, president of Ellison Research, says the youngest ministers seem to have the unhealthiest lifestyles:

The youngest ministers are the heaviest, the most likely to skip meals, the most likely to eat unhealthy foods, the least likely to get exercise, the most likely to go without sufficient sleep, the least likely to take vitamins, the most likely to eat fast food, and the most likely to report problems sleeping. It might be argued that these are eager young ministers out trying to change the world, or at least to build their careers. But it's tragic that they apparently are sacrificing their own health for these purposes. [4]

Health of the Pastor's Family

If you are a family member of a pastor or church staff member, you know only too well the extra pressure that comes with being in the ministry — the high expectations placed on him or her and the hours spent away from the family.

I have several friends who are children of pastors or church staff members. Among them is Ruth, the daughter of a music minister. When she and her sister were in junior high and high school, they formed a group called *"The Ministers' Kids Support Group for Psychiatric Help,"* complete with a constitution, pledge, and actual support group meetings. They invited other pastors' children to it. It was partially a joke, she tells me, but partially not. The pledge began with, "I am a minister's kid. There is absolutely nothing I can do about it!"

Craig Groeschel, senior pastor at LifeChurch.tv, wrote about a lesson he learned from his daughter Catie early in his ministry.

When my first daughter, Catie, was very young, I was the classic overly-driven, ministry-obsessed, type-A personality workaholic. While working full-time as an associate pastor, I was also carrying fifteen hours of seminary classes.

One day I called little Catie on the phone and said I had to stay late at the office to get some work done and would not see her before she went to bed. I promised her I would be home and wake her with a late good night kiss.

Catie innocently said, "Daddy, this is not your home. You live at the office."

I changed my work habits at that moment and have never been the same.[5]

Family Health: Self

- 94 percent agree with the statement, "There is extra pressure being married to a minister," including 54 percent who strongly agree.

- 91 percent agree there is extra pressure being the child of a pastor; 46 percent strongly agree.

- Six out of ten pastors say that their role as a minister prevents them from spending sufficient time with their family.

- On a scale of 1 (extremely unhealthy) to 5 (extremely healthy), pastors were asked to rate the health of their family relationships. The average rating for their relationship with their spouse was 4.5 out of 5, with 47 percent considering their relationship extremely healthy.

- Overall, pastors rated their family health as a 4.

Family Health: View of Other Pastors

- Although pastors give their family relationships high marks (4), when asked to rate the health of other pastors' families, the average rating was 3.2.

- The average minister estimates that 25 percent of pastors he or she knows are having relational issues with a child, and 20 percent of other pastors are having considerable problems in their marriage.

Ellison Research's president Ron Sellers noted the difference between how pastors see their own family health and how they see the health of other clergy families. "Ministers apparently have a much more optimistic view of their own family than they do of the families of other ministers," Sellers stated. "When one out of every twenty ministers feels his or her own family unit is unhealthy, but one out of every seven ministers believes the family units of others in their denomination are unhealthy, there's a disconnect."

Sellers added, "One of these perspectives probably is wrong —either things are not as bad with other ministers' families as the typical pastor believes, or things are not as healthy with their own family as the typical pastor believes."[6]

Based on this research, even if only 5 percent of pastors are in seriously unhealthy relationships with their families, that's almost 20,000 people in the US alone. And that is just an estimate of senior pastors; it doesn't include other church staff workers or volunteers.

Pastors' Satisfaction with Prayer Life

Have you ever read a book that totally wrecked you? For me that book was *Preacher and Prayer* by E. M. Bounds.[7]

In *Preacher and Prayer*, Bounds describes the prayer habits of several Christian men — and not just vocational pastors.

- John Wesley prayed for two hours every morning, starting at 4:00 a.m.

- Edward Payson prayed so often that deep grooves were formed on his hardwood floor by his bedside from where he knelt.

- Abolitionist William Wilberforce spent at least two hours in prayer early in the day.

- John Welch, a Scottish preacher, would think he wasted his day if he spent less than eight to ten hours a day in prayer, sometimes in the middle of the night.

When I first read about these men, I was blown away. To be honest, for me prayer has usually been an afterthought. Or I'd pray when people would request something specific, but I don't think I've ever prayed for probably more than half an hour at a time. And certainly not at 4:00 a.m.! My prayer life was lacking depth. And evidently mine wasn't the only one.

- The average pastor prays 39 minutes a day.

- 21 percent of pastors pray less than 15 minutes a day.

- Those most satisfied with their prayer life spend almost an hour in prayer per day; those who are least satisfied with their prayer life average 21 minutes per day.

- Those most satisfied spend less time making requests and more time being quiet and listening to God; those least satisfied spend a majority of their prayer time making requests.[8]

I realize it's not how long or when you pray that's important. But what was consistent with these men mentioned by Bounds, as well as with several biblical examples — Jacob, David, Daniel, Paul, Jesus — was the sacrifice of their own desires (such as sleep or convenience).

Bounds writes,

> *What the church needs today is not more machinery or better, not new organizations or more and novel methods, but men whom the Holy Ghost can use — men of prayer, men mighty in prayer. The Holy Ghost does not flow through methods, but through men. He does not come on machinery, but on men. He does not anoint plans, but men — men of prayer.*[9]

With prayer being one of the cornerstones of our spiritual disciplines and essential for communion with our Father, it's surprising that such a high number of ministers are not satisfied with their prayer lives.

Casualties of War

It's obvious in the arena of pastors and church leaders that there's a classic battle going on between good and evil. We know what we need to do — to take care of our bodies, our minds, our souls, and our families — but we allow the idol of convenience to replace the knowledge that the Holy Spirit has instilled in us.

Biological warfare has been around for a very long time, but the threats have moved up in our consciousness after September 11, 2001. Terrorists can release lethal biological agents in a small confined space, and because of their careful planning and knowledge of the agent and their target, incurable disease and destruction will rapidly follow.

Satan works in a similar manner. He's been plotting since the fall to ruin mankind, and what better place to start than with the one group of people whose purpose it is to share life with a hurting world. All it takes is infecting one person, and the epidemic can spread like wildfire.

If I were a betting girl, I'd place my money on the fact that almost everyone reading this book has had some type of encounter with a pastor or church leader who has fallen victim to one of the "big three" — sex, money, or power. Almost everybody struggles significantly in at least one of these three areas.

And in worst-case scenarios, you've seen how this person's public struggles have affected more than just the person himself or herself.

My good friend Allen was the lead pastor of a healthy suburban church. For over a dozen years, he had led the church to catch an incredible vision of reaching their local community for Christ. The church had consistently grown for almost twenty years, from about 150 to around 5,000, and had relocated numerous times, most recently into a newly constructed building near several cookie-cutter subdivisions in which working-class dads and soccer moms had taken up residence.

Allen's passion was unquenchable. His heart, worn on his sleeve, was inspiring for anyone who spent time with him. Kimberly, his beautiful wife and mother to his kids, was always seen around the church — involved in the choir, mothers programs, and Bible studies for women.

Allen's "big three" struggle? Sex.

Please don't misunderstand me. I realize we all have our struggles — areas in which Satan tends to home in on with laser-like precision. And no one sin is greater than another. However, with the knowledge of your weaknesses comes the responsibility to protect these areas with the greatest amount of armor possible.

This was the misfortune in Allen's situation. Since he was ashamed of his weakness, he didn't share it with anyone, not even with those who held him accountable. Because Allen believed the lie that nobody would understand his struggle, he also began believing other lies — lies like the one where he was falling in love with another woman, for example.

The constant demands wore down his sense of worth, and with the growth the church was experiencing, more and more people needed to be pleased. After spending hours and hours pouring his life into ministry, doing the work that comes with leading a church, Allen slowly began to drop his guard.

The relationship with the other woman was an escape. What he knew was wrong became twisted into what was right. And he couldn't stop. The on again/off again extramarital affair lasted for years, until one day it couldn't go on anymore. He couldn't lead the church, and he knew it. He was too afraid of being found out. So Allen suddenly tendered his resignation.

God had other plans.

The elder board met with him, asking him to reconsider his position. They told him that if he was stressed-out because of all the new growth, new bills, and new people, they'd give him as much time off as he needed. Allen knew that this wasn't the case. After meeting with the elders for several hours, he confessed.

The elders and leadership team immediately met with church staff members and told them the sad news. Key volunteers were also notified. And the decision was made to announce the resignation to the congregation the following Sunday.

Because of this pastor's prominence in his community, the news hit with the impact of nothing short of a tidal wave. As one of the other pastors read a letter to the church, gasps of shock and sounds of weeping were heard throughout the room. And of course, bad news travels fast. It seemed as though the whole metropolitan area knew before the day was over what had happened, and sadly, most of what was being passed along was simply exaggerated gossip.

People began discussing the situation online. Because of the story's trauma, even those who were unfamiliar with the church and the pastor kept spreading the word. What had first affected just one man now affected thousands of people in one community. And then it turned into epidemic proportions, affecting tens — possibly hundreds — of thousands of people around the world.

A friend of mine spoke with Allen a few days after he had resigned. If his voice was any indication of his soul, Allen's was totally shattered. My friend said that if his and Allen's conversation had been recorded and then mailed to believers everywhere, people would never have affairs again.

Allen was that broken.

Although Allen fell out of God's will, he didn't fall out of God's reach. Allen faced a seemingly impossible restoration. It would take a miracle.

In spite of the terrible pain his decisions caused him, his family, and thousands of people, God picked Allen up, dusted him off, and said, "OK. Now how can we use this for my glory?"

God does the same with us every single day. Seven months into his healing, Allen told me, "There's no doubt I have to live with the consequences. There's no doubt I have a long, long way to go. But grace has never been so real to me. I could preach about grace all day long, but I had never truly experienced it until now."

In Allen's case, there is no doubt that God has his work cut out for him. But isn't that true for all of us?

Code Blue

When a Code Blue is issued in a hospital, any available medical personnel run to the room of the person who is coding. It's a matter of life and death. Milliseconds count. Politics, personal beliefs, hang-ups, grudges, and pride are put aside as the life of a fellow human lies in their hands. It's an emergency.

Since the beginning of time, mankind has been facing a life-and-death emergency. We are separated from our Creator. All he wants is for us to be reconciled to him. He sent his own flesh and blood down to earth to restore us. And we're to help guide others to that restoration.

The greatest commandments are what? To love God and to love our neighbors as we love ourselves. In most cases, I don't question our love for God. The passion and intensity with which we go about our lives are small indicators of our love. But we are guilty of not loving ourselves. The statistics don't lie. And even if they did, I'm sure you could conclude from your own experience that, quite frankly, we're pretty terrible at loving ourselves.

If we can't love ourselves, we can't love others in the way that God has designed us. We can care for others and can want the best for them, but to love them in the godliest way is impossible until we can obey this great commandment.

We are in the midst of a crisis that needs our full devotion of mind, body, and spirit.

In Mark 12:30, Jesus declares, "Love the Lord your God with all your heart and with all your soul and with all your mind and with all your strength."

Notice Jesus doesn't tell us to "love others with all your strength"; he says to "love the Lord your God." By loving God, we're faithful to his commandments. And when we're obedient, God will carry out his work through us. He will prepare us for battle in all areas.

Satan is out to annihilate hope and light, both in our world and in us, the body of Christ. He's well aware of the crisis of the human race, and he will do anything and everything in his power to obliterate our efforts.

As the church, we need to take a good, hard look around and ask ourselves if we are ready to fight. To fight for our own love relationship with God through Christ, and for the world around us as well.

Second Opinion

Perry Noble, senior pastor,
NewSpring Church, Anderson, South Carolina

A. M. M.: What are some things you do to help you recognize when you need a breather?

P. N.: One of the first things I do is try to listen to my body. Whenever I catch myself with that tired feeling for more than two or three days, I know that rest is much needed.

Also I try to pay attention to how tolerant I am of other people. If I find myself getting upset at even the most trivial thing, it's time to break away for a while.

And finally, when I begin to think, "I just can't do this anymore," or, "I really wish I didn't have to preach this weekend," then I know that being stressed and tired are the sources of that line of thinking, because thinking that way goes against the calling that Jesus has placed on my life.

A. M. M.: When you struggle with something negative that you're having a hard time shaking, where do you turn?

P. N.: I have to honestly say that this question is something I am continually wrestling with and struggling through.

First of all, I really do find comfort and encouragement in the Scriptures. Also I turn to the team I serve with. They are able to help me see that, though the situation seems to be enormous and out of control, it is actually all in God's hands.

A. M. M.: When a disease is contagious, it can spread quickly and infect others. How do you combat mad church disease in your church?

P. N.: One of the things I've always done is directly confront any blatant untruths that are being said about the ministry God has given us. I usually do it in a humorous way, and in doing so, I've actually given the people in our church both ammunition and permission to confront untruthful things in love.

A. M. M.: Cows don't have a chance when it comes to surviving mad cow disease. Thankfully for us, one of God's favorite things to do is to restore our relationship with him and with others. When things look hopeless and God seems far away, what are some truths you meditate on?

P. N.: I meditate on the fact that he has called me into ministry, that he is sovereign and is not surprised by anything, that Jesus Christ endured way more than I will ever endure and he never quit, and so I shouldn't either. I think about how I feel, and I think about what is real — and they are often two separate things. I think about how God has given me the Holy Spirit to guide me through all situations — and God promises us life.

PART 2

AM I AT RISK?

EXAMINING RISK FACTORS

AND SYMPTOMS

Chapter 4: Internal Risk Factors

You have got to be kidding me," I said to my doctor. "I'm only twenty-seven. I'm totally healthy!"

I was at my annual physical — or better to say, my once-a-decade physical. I hadn't had a full workup with my family practitioner since I was sixteen.

He rolled back on his little doctor's stool and flipped through my chart.

"I really do think you should have an EKG, just to be on the safe side. There are heart problems on both sides of your family, and especially with what your dad's been through and the fact that you seem to overload yourself — well, I just think it'd be a good idea."

I couldn't argue. He had been our family doctor for well over a decade and knew that my dad had had quintuple bypass heart surgery three years prior. And he had seen me through all my stressful ups and downs.

I let the nurse apply a dozen or so little suction cups to my body and get a readout of my heart's rhythms.

"Well, it looks like everything's good," the nurse said, and my doctor confirmed it.

I walked out of the exam room to a waiting room full of people three times my age, waiting to get their own tickers checked.

I felt ridiculous as I passed them. But at the same time, I secretly appreciated my doctor's initiative. He knew I could have a genetic predisposition for heart problems, and he wanted to make sure we were being proactive with my health.

(Interesting update: I first wrote this book in 2007 when I was 27. Now, as I edit this, I'm 34 and I've had to have two heart surgeries to correct a genetic arrhythmia I developed called super ventricular tachycardia – or SVT. I've been symptom-free for two years, so all should be well. It's just interesting how things do change over time!)

In order to get a good understanding of mad church disease, we've got to take a look at our health from every angle, starting at the beginning.

Are certain kinds of people more likely to experience burnout? Does burnout happen because of our environment?

Taking a look back at my doctor's decision to run an EKG, I can tell he looked at both internal and external factors. Internally, he knew I had a family history of heart issues.

Externally, he knew I often overcommitted myself, which could lead to unnecessary strain on my heart. Those two facts alone are significant risk factors for developing heart problems, even at an early age.

In the same vein, both internal and external factors contribute to mad church disease.

Certain internal factors can make us more at risk for becoming burned out. Most of these are features we are born with. They reflect how God knit together the fibers of our being. And because they are fairly hard-wired, these characteristics aren't easily changed, and that is OK. We have to accept the fact that, although these may sometimes seem like limitations, they are the very things that make us unique.

Personality Type

Most of us are familiar with type A and type B personality descriptors.[1]

Look at the table on the next page.

Which personality type do you lean toward?

You may have both type A and type B characteristics, but you probably have a clear view of your dominant personality type.

Type A Characteristics	Type B Characteristics
Impatient / Time conscious	Patient
Concerned about status	Relaxed
Competitive	Easygoing
Aggressive	Creative
Incapable of relaxing	Imaginative
Easily able to multitask	Self-analytical
Shows workaholic tendencies	Often described as laid-back

The general assumption is that type A personalities tend to burn out easier than type B, but it's not always the case.

Dean was a really casual kind of guy. He pastored a church in a small community — and he preferred to. His gentle demeanor was a stunning reflection of Christ, and his patience seemed endless. Although he was a great communicator, it wasn't because he had a charismatic personality. When he spoke, you had to listen. Every word was well thought out and inspiring. Because of his creative and easygoing personality, he was always thinking of new ways to reach people for Christ. And he had no problem with relaxing. You could find him early on Saturday mornings fishing in a nearby river with other men from the neighborhood.

It's pretty obvious Dean was a classic type B. He wasn't concerned about status. He was laid-back and imaginative. But because of his patience and easygoing personality, he had a very difficult time saying no.

Dean's burnout began very slowly. A few church members would drop by the parsonage unannounced. He would show them in, serve coffee and dessert, and patiently listen to their problems. What started out with a couple of people stopping in a couple of times a month turned into several members stopping by multiple times a week.

Dean's strengths of being sensitive and friendly also became his weaknesses. Because he didn't know how to set boundaries, his approach began handicapping him. Soon Dean's bucket became empty. He no longer had the energy to minister to others in the way he knew was necessary. His growing ineffectiveness triggered a depression, and he eventually left the ministry.

Dean took time off. He relaxed. He didn't continually go a hundred miles an hour. Yet Dean still burned out.

On the flip side, Janelle is a type A. She's a busy mom and wife who also works part-time in health care. Her husband travels frequently, and her sons, ages seventeen and twelve, are active in school and church activities.

Janelle has never received a paycheck from her church, but she's there several times a week. She serves on the worship team, making sure everyone is in the correct place at the correct time. She participates in the creative team planning for all the services. If there's a broken piece between the original brainstorming session and the execution of the service, Janelle will be the first to step up and fix it.

Her driven personality is essential for her volunteer role. God has gifted her to be organized and strategic, as well as energetic and full of a "Let's go get 'em, tiger!" attitude.

After three years of dutiful, dedicated service, Janelle called the media pastor and quit out of the blue. It was right before the Christmas season — and with her oldest son due to graduate in a few months, the stress of volunteer service on top of family responsibilities was just too much. Soon, Janelle wasn't seen around the church at all. Even though the media pastor would occasionally call to check in, Janelle faded away. She had burned out.

Like Dean, because Janelle didn't know how to manage her strength as a type A personality, it eventually became her Achilles' heel and took her out of the game.

Our History

Another internal influence for developing mad church disease is our past, which is as unique as our personality. Our family structures as children, our education, and our spiritual journeys have an effect on how we see our lives today and on how we plan our future. Deeply rooted trauma or habitual choices made over time make us more inclined to act in certain ways. We still make our own decisions, but our past is what makes us distinct.

Take Cindy, for example. Growing up, she always earned good grades in school. Her parents encouraged her to participate in extracurricular activities, so she played sports, participated in the Spanish club, and helped mentor other students.

What Cindy was unable to realize at the time was the power her parents' expectations had over her. As long as she stayed on the honor roll and kept her social calendar full, they were happy. However, once her grades dropped, they expressed their disappointment. She decided to limit some of her activities to focus on her studies, but her parents became frustrated that she wasn't performing at a level acceptable to them.

Fast-forward fifteen years. Cindy now works as the volunteer women's director in her church. She also serves in the children's ministry and occasionally sings in the choir. Her parents no longer have an active influence on her decision-making, but their impact still rings loud and clear.

Growing up, Cindy lived in a constant state of fear. She was afraid that if her perfect balance of school and extracurricular activities unraveled, her parents would be right there to let her know. And now that she's active in her church, the same fear of disappointment controls her emotions and behaviors around the clock.

Instead of trying to appease her parents, she tries to appease her ministry leader. She often takes work home with her, staying connected to her phone and email at all times. If something comes up, she doesn't want to let the ball drop. She's afraid that if she unplugs for even a moment, she'll be letting her team down.

Maybe you didn't receive much affirmation growing up, so you run yourself ragged trying to please others and fill that gaping hole you carry around. Or maybe one of your parents left, which put you in a position of having to be responsible at a young age — and now you can't let it go as an adult. So you're taking responsibility for others to make things work right. Perhaps you were traumatized or abused, and the only way you can numb the pain is to fill your life with busyness. That's what I did.

As much as we may want to, we can never rid ourselves of our past — the good or the bad. And regardless of how normal or how terrible your past may have been, you've experienced it all for a reason. The successes, the failures, the joy, and the pain are all beautifully woven together to make you who you are at this moment.

We should look at our past as a gift and not a burden. And as such, we should steward it like any other gift we've been given. We need to be grateful for our unique circumstances, not resentful. Once we accept our God-given past, we can find out what about it makes us extraordinary. How can we channel a propensity toward responsibility — as in Cindy's case? How can we encourage others who have a past similar to ours?

By taking our focus off the dysfunctions of our past, and changing it to how God can work through us as he uses our life journey — our history, our present, and our future — we are less likely to burn out. Any time we become less and God becomes more, it's his power being perfected in us.

Our Health

Our physical health impacts our day-to-day living more than we may realize. From our sleep habits to the way we eat or even exercise, our health can influence our susceptibility to burn out.

When I lived in Dallas, I got to know a pastor named Joe. Just a few weeks after meeting him, while I was doing some communication consulting with his church, Joe fell off the face of the earth.

With nothing but a short email telling me he would be away from the church for a few months, he directed me to another staff member. I wondered what had happened to Joe. Several months later, he contacted me and told me that his leadership team had forced him to take two months off from ministry. He was on the brink of total exhaustion.

The symptoms manifested in several ways — mostly a mixture of physical and spiritual effects. And his physical stress, compounded by a seething anger, had gotten to a point where it nearly killed him.

One easy way you can be taken down fast is by simply not taking care of yourself. The areas in your health you neglect now will eventually catch up to you. In Joe's case, it took almost an entire decade of ignoring the warning signs. We're given one shot at taking care of our bodies, and it's our decision whether we'll take the information available to us to make wise choices. Or we can ignore it — and burn out.

Our Relationship with Christ

Last, but certainly most important, is the way in which we walk with Christ in our daily relationship with him. Are we walking in such a way that the Spirit guides each and every step, or are we finding things to do and asking God only to bless our efforts?

The biblical story of David shows the indescribable closeness that comes when we humbly seek God and rely on his power, as well as the tragedy that inevitably strikes when we stray.

From the moment David was anointed to be king of Israel in 1 Samuel 16, it was obvious to those around him that God was with him. When one of Saul's attendants suggested that they find a harpist to help relieve the distress an evil spirit was causing Saul, another servant suggested David: "I have seen a son of Jesse of Bethlehem who knows how to play the harp. He is a brave man and a warrior. He speaks well and is a fine-looking man. *And the LORD is with him*" (1 Samuel 16:18, emphasis mine).

Later, David reappears when Goliath and the Philistines are challenging the Israelites. Even though it didn't make sense that a young man should take on a nine-foot giant, Saul agrees to let David go, saying, "The LORD be with you" (1 Samuel 17:37).

When all David should have wanted to do was run, he stood his ground against Goliath:

> *David said to the Philistine, "You come against me with sword and spear and javelin, but I come against you in the name of the LORD Almighty, the God of the armies of Israel, whom you have defied. This day the LORD will hand you over to me, and I'll strike you down and cut off your head. Today I will give the carcasses of the Philistine army to the birds of the air and the beasts of the earth, and the whole world will know that there is a God in Israel."*
>
> — 1 Samuel 17:45–46

David had no armor. He had his past. God had given him experience fighting lions and bears as a shepherd. And God had given David the confidence he needed to go out "in the name of the LORD Almighty." In verse 46, David expresses that he knows — beyond a shadow of a doubt — that God will hand over Goliath to him so that David can finish him off. David clearly says it's not because of his strength, or even his weapons, that Goliath will fall.

It is simply because of God.

David's belief that God would deliver on his promises was all he needed. Not for one moment when faced with Goliath and the Philistines did David buckle under the pressure. He never ran from it. The Bible never says he was even afraid; in fact, it suggests just the opposite: "As the Philistine moved closer to attack him, David ran quickly toward the battle line to meet him" (1 Samuel 17:48).

David ran quickly toward the battle line.

There are certainly times in our spiritual journeys when we feel that same fresh passion. We feel reckless because we are walking (or running) completely in God's power.

After David became king of Israel, he received a message from God through the prophet Nathan, reminding him of God's faithfulness in the past and God's desire to make a covenant with him for the future.

Throughout David's reign as king, he goes to war many, many times. He wins battle after battle. He blesses the house of Saul. He rules over Israel. Needless to say, David's a pretty busy guy. And over the course of time, he slowly begins to stray from God's perfect plan.

In 2 Samuel 11, it's springtime. Instead of spending time standing in awe of the budding trees and listening to the harmonies of the singing birds, the kings in that era went off to war. David was no exception. Even though he personally stayed in Jerusalem, he sent out armies to destroy the Ammonites. We all know the story. David sees the beautiful Bathsheba bathing. He wants her. He gets her. They even conceived a child together.

Big oops.

Remember how David earlier had run toward the battle line to defeat Goliath? I'm pretty sure he was running hard and fast the other way now to get out of this mess. He tells lies. He deceives his men. He devises a plan. He orders Uriah (Bathsheba's husband) home and gets him drunk so he'll sleep with his wife.

Maybe they could pass the pregnancy off as what happened as a result of that encounter.

But it didn't work. Uriah was so devoted to his army that he turns down the offer of "special privileges." He refuses to sleep with Bathsheba while his men are still out fighting.

I can see David pacing the floor wondering how to take care of this situation. The only possible solution he saw was to kill Uriah.

And that's what happened. David makes a plan and sets Uriah up to die on the battle line. Not only did Uriah die, but also other men in his army were killed in the fight. David continues to cover up his tracks by telling more and more lies. And for the first time in the Bible's account of David's life, it no longer says that the LORD was with him.

Instead, 2 Samuel 11:27 tells us, "But the thing David had done displeased the LORD."

We all make mistakes. We all screw up. And it doesn't mean that God leaves us. David wasn't perfect before meeting Bathsheba. But we can learn several things from his story.

We have a choice of what we keep in front of us: We can either keep our eyes focused on what God can accomplish through his power in our lives or choose to focus on what I call "the dangerous distractions."

When we are walking in step with God and in his power, he places his favor on us. Others notice that God is working in and through us. We, on the other hand, are completely oblivious to the intensity with which God is using us.

However, when we focus on the dangerous distractions, God simply won't stand for it. He offers his forgiveness, his mercy, and hope, to be sure, but we must confess and fall back on his strength before we move forward on the journey he has laid out for each of us.

Chapter 5: External Risk Factors

Although many internal factors can predispose us to experience burnout, certain things within our environment — external factors, in other words — when not handled appropriately, can influence our decisions negatively.

Tools of Our Tools

When I first started working in ministry, I had your everyday, ordinary cell phone. It placed and received calls, and that was pretty much it. Over time, and by my own free will, I've upgraded to the Smartphone. It emails. It sends texts. It checks the score of the Dallas Mavericks games. It wakes me up at 5:30 every morning and let's me snooze twice for ten minutes at a time. It keeps my calendar and gives me directions and lets me play games – I mean, do my taxes.

Can I be honest?

For a while my phone owned my life.

I lost control.

This fact actually struck me one day in the shower. I was getting ready to go to one of the weekend services when I was on a church staff and I had an idea about a project. So, since my phone was already in the bathroom (you know, just in case someone needed me), I actually started sending emails and text messages from the shower!

We always make fun of people who talk on their phones in the bathroom, or how unsanitary it is for people to use them to text or email while they're, how shall we delicately say it, "taking care of business" — but I really think I crossed a sad, sad line when I couldn't wait for five minutes and felt like I needed to send those messages right then and there from the shower.

That is a lack of control.

I confessed my shower email-sending episode to a friend (and now to you — how embarrassing!) I mean, really. Some things need to be left sacred.

Technology is a powerful tool, but as Henry David Thoreau once wrote, "Men have become the tools of their tools." In 2008, I spent some time in Africa with Compassion International. We visited several projects where even the most primitive forms of technology did not exist. If we weren't in a hotel or restaurant, more than likely our bathroom was a hole cut in the ground.

One of the visions of our time in Africa was to have the trip participants, who were all bloggers, document in video, photography, and words what we saw and felt. Fifteen different perspectives reaching fifteen different audiences, all for the common goal of releasing children from poverty in Jesus' name.

Before the trip, organizers carefully researched the hotels in Kampala, Uganda, where we would be staying, so that Internet access would be guaranteed and we'd be able to blog consistently from Uganda. However, things didn't go as planned.

Our Internet service, if it worked, was slow at best (it took me an hour once to upload four small photos). Many of our cell phones didn't have international plans, so calling our families back home was also out of the question. The first few days I felt phantom alerts until I remembered that my phone had no signal in the middle of Africa.

No phone connections and sporadic Internet use forced the fifteen of us to disconnect in a way that probably none of us had ever done before.

Honestly, I think most of us were frustrated for the first few days —
mainly because we were unable to share what we were experiencing with our readers. What's more, the inability to connect with our families and friends back home made us feel even more disconnected.

It is difficult to unplug. Internet is relatively inexpensive, as are mobile phones that connect us to social media and email. Our TVs and various TV subscription services and tablets and now, even our watches, give us comfort and convenience, but when we rely on them so heavily, they also give us headaches and no time for solitude.

Lack of Control

I know from my own experience as a preacher's kid, as well as from my time spent in ministry, that we often feel as though we don't have a choice in what we do or don't do. How many times have you said, "If I don't take care of this, it's never going to get done"? We assume the pressure is on us (and it very well might be), and as a result, we slowly begin to lose control over our thinking, and then over our behavior.

Aside from our phone/email/internet/text addictions, other things can make us feel out of control. Sometimes we don't get to choose what our tasks are, and we're stuck doing something we're not passionate about. Sometimes we're constrained by financial challenges or a lack of other resources. Maybe the hours we're required to work are out of our control and becoming a pressure in the life we have outside of the office.

Pressure to Be the Best

We are creatures who need affirmation. And the spotlight seems to promise us everything we've ever wanted. Whether it's an actual spotlight on the platform in front of an adoring congregation or a more passive spotlight — perhaps you glow under the praise of a certain leader — it's natural to seek out opportunities in which we can shine and be at our best.

One of the problems I see plaguing unhealthy environments is ego. Ego can show itself as loud and abrasive, or as subtle and deceiving. Either way, it's the antithesis of the character of Christ.

Society today is competitive. We feel that our voices must be the loudest and carry the furthest in order to be heard and validated. It breaks my heart when I hear pastors of small churches say, "We only had seventy-five people today" or "Only two hundred people showed up."

Only? I'm sorry. Are those seventy-five or two hundred people not enough for you?

I'm not going to discuss at length the perceived importance of numbers. Keeping track of "how many" is usually a valid metric to measure an aspect of effectiveness in terms of what we are doing. Numbers do represent people. Jesus did say that he would build his church. However, we don't always have such a clear view of what this looks like in our churches today.

Unfortunately, I think numbers have become an addiction. We flaunt our numbers, despise our numbers, and fret about our numbers. Our numbers validate us. But they shouldn't. We often don't know how God is using us. We only need to know that he is — and respond with grateful hearts.

This spirit of competitiveness (whether overtly stated or merely implied) has damaged so many churches and leaders who haven't seen the same "success." After hearing it over and over, leaders who aren't as "successful" start believing the lies that maybe God just hasn't blessed them like he "blesses" other churches or leaders. And at that point, those leaders either shut down or begin to be driven by their need for affirmation.

When we think that our calling is to be the biggest, the most creative, or the best, we have completely lost sight of the only important fact.

We are called.

Let me clarify. There is nothing wrong with competition. There is nothing wrong with passionately wanting to show the love of Jesus to as many people as possible. And there is certainly nothing wrong with celebrating.

If you know that you're a competitive leader, I highly encourage you to seek some honest feedback from those you are leading. You may be creating an environment of unhealthy competition, driven by your own desire to succeed instead of by God's desire to work through you.

Paul writes to the Philippians about this kind of unity through humility:

> *If you have any encouragement from being united with Christ, if any comfort from his love, if any fellowship with the Spirit, if any tenderness and compassion, then make my joy complete by being like-minded, having the same love, being one in spirit and purpose. Do nothing out of selfish ambition or vain conceit, but in humility consider others better than yourselves.*
>
> — Philippians 2:1 – 3

How often do we consider others better than ourselves? My experience is that it's really easy to trash-talk churches or methods that aren't what we think they should be. What is troubling is how easily I've done this and how often I've seen it done.

When I take time to reflect, I feel a vast amount of conviction about conversations I've been a part of where we've grumbled about this person, this ministry, and this church. How desensitized many of us have become!

These rants (both subtle and obvious) litter our everyday conversations, blog posts, and emails. And if we are so vocally open about them, what is truly the condition of our hearts with regard to unity?

A healthy environment is formed in the spirit of true humility.

It's humility that causes us to want to step out of the spotlight and take ourselves out of the picture.

It's humility that makes us desire to sacrifice our own need for affirmation and acknowledgment and to bring fame and glory only to the One who made us.

It's humility that not only puts God first but puts others in front of us as well.

Unclear Expectations

Adam was new to the children's team. In fact, his position was entirely new. With the rapid growth that his church's children's ministry had experienced, he hit the ground running, implementing new ideas into the children's worship services and overseeing a team of volunteers.

Because Adam jumped in so quickly, nobody really ever gave him any expectations for his position. At first, Adam thought that the lack of communication indicated a level of trust in him, and he took that responsibility and promised not to let anyone down. However, over time, Adam realized that he didn't know what his boundaries were — when it was OK to say yes or no.

The lack of clear expectations caused Adam to take a "better safe than sorry" approach to his position. He said yes to almost every opportunity that came along. Soon, Adam's wife began to notice how much time he was spending at the church on weekends. She wanted to talk to him about his being away from home so much, but she didn't want to make him feel guilty. After all, it was a relatively rare experience for Adam to discover something he really enjoyed. So she kept quiet most of the time.

Without clear communication coming from his leadership team at church, Adam began to feel overwhelmed by the tasks he faced. Was he expected to complete them all? How would he find resources to complete them? Who should he talk to in order to get the appropriate permission? And at home, he wasn't sure what his wife was expecting. He began to feel as if he was walking on eggshells.

After one particularly stressful weekend, Adam came home. His wife, who was upset because of the amount of time he had been spending at church, laid a guilt trip on him. The combination of the weekend and the tension at home caused Adam to snap. He was just a heartbeat away from calling in and quitting when he took a step back and a deep breath — and began to evaluate the situation.

Adam and his wife openly discussed what his ideal schedule would look like. And he communicated to his colleagues at church that on certain nights, he wouldn't be available.

Instead of waiting for someone else to lay out expectations for him, Adam took the initiative to put those boundaries in place so others would know what to expect from him.

Communication is essential when it comes to setting and meeting expectations. Sometimes we don't know what our leaders expect from us. Do we have the authority to take on that new project? Can we spend that money? Just when are we expected to be serving, and when can we take time to be refreshed and reequipped?

Conflicts in Personality or Values

Working in ministry can prove to have explosive results if we don't share key values with our team. We can work through the smaller differences, but if we aren't on the same page with regard to key issues, we put both our teams and ourselves at risk for burning out.

A micromanaging supervisor or even a gossipy coworker can put stress on your performance. Over time, this stress can build up until you shut down and stop performing. If you're on staff at a church that places a high value on financial responsibility and stewardship, but you don't think twice about spending money on the first thing that crosses your desk, you could be in trouble. Or maybe you care deeply about reaching the children in your community, but your church wants to reach only senior citizens. The cumulative effect of the stress caused by these differences can lead to burnout.

Mismatch of Job Skills/Passions

I am not what you'd call a numbers person. For me to work on budgets and finances — anything really to do with money — is a hard task. Fortunately, as an author, a very small amount of time is spent playing with a calculator and a spreadsheet. I still have to do expense reports, figure out budgets, and plan how much to spend for each year, but these tasks are few and far between. Tim and I are fortunate enough to have a friend who eats, sleeps, and breathes numbers and helps us out with that kind of work. He loves it! If you put me in his shoes for a day, I'd lose my mind because I don't have the required skills, nor do I have the passion for it.

Skills can only get you so far. It takes heart to fulfill your purpose the way God intends it to be fulfilled.

Old-School Church Politics

A new pastor, fresh out of seminary, took his first position as a pastor of a church. He gathered the elders to discuss the church's plans for the upcoming year. With each suggestion, he was met with the words, "Well, that's not the way we've done it before." Instead of letting this response cause tension, the pastor simply moved down his list until by the end of the meeting, he realized that not one thing he had suggested would be implemented.

Even though he didn't like to cause trouble, he did bring up the fact that they did ask him to lead and direct the church. He was answered with the following:

"My grandfather helped build this church!"

"My mother sang in this church's choir for fifteen years!"

"Our family has been tithing here since before you were born!"

Resistance to trying new things is a large stress factor for those in the church. Transitioning a church full of people who have been happy in their pews for forty years is a well-nigh insurmountable problem.

New-School Church Politics

A church doesn't have to be well established in order for it to be full of politics. Sometimes even the newest churches are filled with big visions — and equally large egos. The passion of a church planter is unmistakable. Without careful guidance and mentoring from those who have walked that road before, the church leadership team can turn into a "good ole boys" club, with the pastor leading the pack and his closest friends making all the decisions. In this scenario, there's likely no diversity and no proper confrontation or accountability. When increasing demands require the church to take on new staff or seek additional help, the new people often feel out of place and pressured to fulfill someone else's dream for them instead of the one God has given them.

No Freedom to Dream

Early in my ministry, a pastor told me something that would forever change my outlook on dreaming. After we had met to talk about how my God-given dreams could fit into my role in the church, he looked at me and said, "Anne, your dreams are just too big for our church. Maybe it's time you found somewhere else you can dream."

Even though I was heartbroken, gradually I became inspired to prove him right. I know God's plans are way beyond what I can even imagine, so I want my dreams to be too big!

I realize that many of you have experienced something similar. You've been full of passion for something God has given you, only to have it shot down. You've faced the tension of figuring out how to respect those in authority over you — or to believe in your heart that those in authority should get out of the way. Maybe you are the leader, and other staff members aren't supporting you. Maybe you're being undermined. What do you do? Do you leave? Do you stay and work to be an influence?

What if you dream, and that dream dies in the hands of someone else? You begin to lose the courage to process these providential ideas, and soon, it's just easier to carry out your mundane day-to-day tasks in order to avoid getting hurt again. Even though my broken dream occurred several years ago, I still find myself extremely hesitant when it comes to expressing the things I'm most passionate about. When you've experienced this kind of hurt, it affects the way you think and dream about God, people, and especially your role in the church.

The Furnace

Being in ministry, you've never had any irrational thoughts, have you? You've never wanted to shove that annoying worship leader off the stage or shake that parent who thinks her child just has to be with the grade school children because he is so much smarter than those other kids in kindergarten. You've never wanted to tell your pastor off because the church has consumed all of your husband's time and now he's missed your first child's first words, first steps, and, oh my, her first date.

No, you've never had those thoughts. Because being a Christian is all about the hugs and giggles. We're smiles all the time, right?

Here's the reality: there is no perfect environment out there.

There are no perfect churches to serve in, no perfect pastors to work for, and no perfect environments.

And generally speaking, most people you run into in the church world are great, loving, caring people.

Stop laughing.

But I'm going to guess that more than half of you reading this at least smirked at that "great, loving, caring" line. Why?

Because you've been there — where it's not great.

Or loving.

Or caring.

At all.

And because of that, see how easy it is to be cynical?

(Says the pot to the kettle — trust me, I'm working on this one too.)

. . .

Being placed in a tough environment isn't something new. Around 600 BC, four gentlemen by the names of Daniel, Shadrach, Meshach, and Abednego were given positions as servants to the Babylonian government.

At first, the training they had to go through didn't seem too bad. Eat food from the king's table. Drink the king's wine. After indulging themselves for three years, they'd be ready to serve the king.

Seriously. Sign me up!

However, the men refuse the king's delicacies, probably because of the strict laws that defined what was historically "clean" and "unclean" as far as food went in that culture. This decision could have terrible consequences for the men.

Daniel tries to negotiate with one of the officials, who is worried that these Israelites' denial of the king's order will cost him his own life. But Daniel reassures him and makes the official a deal:

> *"Please test your servants for ten days: Give us nothing but vegetables to eat and water to drink. Then compare our appearance with that of the young men who eat the royal food, and treat your servants in accordance with what you see." So he agreed to this and tested them for ten days.*
> — Daniel 1:12 – 14

Daniel has faith in God despite unfavorable circumstances — he, along with Shadrach, Meshach, and Abednego, could have been killed for not eating what the king provided.

Yet God is in control.

And after the ten-day test, the four men prove to be stronger and smarter than those who had followed the king's orders — and they gain favor with the king.

Fast-forward a bit, and things start heating up for Shadrach, Meshach, and Abednego.

King Nebuchadnezzar decides to make an idol — a ninety-foot-tall golden idol. At the dedication of this huge statue, a proclamation is shouted out that anyone who doesn't worship the idol will be thrown into a furnace.

Well, the Ten Commandments, which Shadrach, Meshach, and Abednego followed as immutable law, clearly state, "You shall have no other gods before me." They know they have to be obedient to God in spite of their circumstance — even if it brings them to the point of death.

Being confronted by the king and later thrown into a fiery furnace as punishment doesn't sound like the most comfortable place to be, now, does it?

The king learns of the refusal of Shadrach, Meshach, and Abednego to follow his order. And he gets pretty ticked. The Bible describes Nebuchadnezzar as "furious with rage" (Daniel 3:13).

I love that intensity — the king was furious with rage.

And the three men — well, they tell Nebuchadnezzar that their God is strong enough to save them from the fire if they are thrown into the blazing furnace.

This is some serious faith. These three guys are about to be tossed into fire. Real, live, red-hot fire. And yet they are absolutely certain of God's sovereignty over the situation — God's sovereignty over their environment.

Their calm answer does nothing to appease the king. Instead, he gets even more fired up. He orders the furnace to be heated seven times hotter and has the strongest soldiers tie up the men.

It isn't long before the king becomes puzzled.

First, the Bible says the men fell into the furnace. I'm going to do my best here and assume that this isn't a tiny oven. If the king built a ninety-foot idol, who knows how big his death machine is.

Then, much to his surprise, he sees four men walking around in the furnace. The idea of any men walking around is crazy enough. They are tied up. The fire is HOT. The fall itself was probably enough to kill a man.

And then there's this fourth guy?

The fourth man appears to be some kind of heavenly being. The king walks over to the furnace and tells the men to come out. They do, and they are completely unharmed. They don't even smell like smoke. God has completely protected them from the blazing fire.

• • •

In ministry, we spend a lot of time in uncomfortable places. Sometimes we stand up for what we believe in, and we get shot down; sometimes we believe we're truly listening to and following God's call — and despite our best efforts, we often end up in our own fiery furnaces.

Will we trust God in the place we find ourselves? How do we trust God in these external circumstances?

Case Study: John's Furnace

John is someone who's been through the fire. A former executive pastor, he shared his story with me:

> I've worked in state government, a Fortune 500 company, and even a political campaign. The worst experience I've ever had at a job was working in full-time ministry. What makes this more ironic is that I raised my own salary support for the job too, so this church didn't even have to pay me.
>
> The mood around the office was very tense. If you messed up, you heard about it in staff meeting. Arguments were pretty frequent, and the majority of staff thrived on conflict. However, when you're someone who doesn't enjoy conflict, it made for a very tough environment.
>
> I was told in my interview process that family was a high priority.

However, I would be reprimanded when I would occasionally take an extended lunch to attend one of my children's activities. It got to the point where my job was eventually threatened after I stayed home to care for my sick child. I hadn't been absent frequently — just twice in a six-month period.

Did I mention that I raised my own support? The threat of being fired from a job you weren't getting paid for was very difficult to deal with.

Besides the tension, it was one of the most morally uncomfortable environments I had ever worked in. The subject of sex was discussed on an almost daily basis. Staff discussed sexual positions, who in the church was "hot," who in your small group you would have sex with, if two women having sex was considered "hot," and even compared the length of a certain part of the male anatomy.

It went far beyond "guy" talk. I had never encountered that type of conversation in my career, and I have worked for some interesting people.

When I first read John's story, I was angry, sad, mortified, and extremely heartbroken. Even though I had been embroiled in some turbulent church conflicts before, nothing to my knowledge was ever publicly discussed in such a frank and unbiblical manner.

To have pastors — shepherds of a church — sharing in such an inappropriate manner was shocking to me (and being a PK, not much surprises me!), and honestly, it is just really, really creepy.

And to have your job (which you've raised your own support for) threatened for taking care of your family? Absurd — yet far too common in the church world. I know John isn't the only person out there who's heard this threat.

I emailed John back almost immediately and asked him to share more of his story. How did he survive such a terrible environment?

John wrote me back:

This entire situation shook my belief in God and the church to the core. I would love to say that I did everything right and that I voiced concerns about inappropriate activities at every turn. Instead, I remained quiet most of the time. I didn't think that expressing concerns would do any good. I was afraid that it would just worsen my situation.

My prayer life faltered, and my relationship with God wore down. I sunk into a deep depression, and I really had no connection with anyone. I was just a zombie. Finally out of desperation, I emailed a counselor friend of mine and started going to therapy. We continued to meet, and I realized that the depression I was feeling was really anger I had been burying deep inside about this situation at the church.

I did not feel that I had a voice, and when I did voice things, I felt they were ignored or dismissed. It has taken a great deal of work for me to get better. I quit the job, went through therapy, took an antidepressant, and really leaned on the support of my family.

Work, prayer, support, and a strong foundation of faith, family, and friends were the only things that have brought me through this. There are so many times when friends I spoke to were given the right words to say to me at that time. They also encouraged me in the direction that I should go so that I could heal. I could have prayed to be healed from depression, but if I hadn't taken the necessary steps, I would have never come out of it.

I don't have all the answers as to why things happened or were allowed to happen. I really came out of this with more questions than answers. However, I do realize one thing. Just because a church is growing in numbers doesn't mean it is a healthy church. If you're in an abusive environment, get out! Just because the environment is a church is no excuse to stay.

I've also realized who I really work for. I work for God. One thing I discovered when I was able to break away from the situation was that I never worked for the lead pastor. I was working for God. In the end, it is God to whom I'm accountable.

A Blaze of Glory

Even through the fire — through the tension, the conflict, the depression, and the stress — we need to recognize that God is and always has been completely in control. Even through the most difficult circumstances, we become able to share his story, to share his healing, and to give glory to God, which is what it's all about anyway.

You may be in a great place right now. If that's the case, look around you and see who might be going through a fire. Walk alongside them. Pray for them. On the flip side, you may be right in the middle of the furnace. Reflect back on God's faithfulness throughout Scripture. His hand is over your life. As difficult as it may be, pray for wisdom in how to rejoice within your circumstances.

The apostle Paul was probably one of the most persecuted believers in history: "I have worked much harder, been in prison more frequently, been flogged more severely, and been exposed to death again and again" (2 Corinthians 11:23).

From what Paul wrote in 2 Corinthians 11, he seemed to experience many of the same things experienced by those who serve in ministry.

> *Three times I was beaten with rods, once I was stoned, three times I was shipwrecked, I spent a night and a day in the open sea* (OK, that probably hasn't happened to most of us), *I have been constantly on the move* (check). *I have been in danger from rivers, in danger from bandits, in danger from my own countrymen, in danger from Gentiles; in danger in the city, in danger in the country, in danger at sea* (check*); and in danger from false brothers* (check, check). *I have labored and toiled and have often gone without sleep* (check); *I have known hunger and thirst and have often gone without food* (check); *I have been cold and naked* (we'll just say cold here, OK?). *Besides everything else, I face daily the pressure of my concern for all the churches* (Wow! Don't we all?!). *Who is weak, and I do not feel weak? Who is led into sin, and I do not inwardly burn* (Now we're really talking!)?
>
> — 2 Corinthians 11:25 – 29, commentary added

I'm sure many of us can relate to the things Paul carried on his shoulders. What's a person to do? Most of us would cry out to God and ask for these problems to be removed or resolved. We'd ask for protection from these circumstances — or more likely for deliverance!

Even throughout his many imprisonments, even when faced with death, Paul sent letters to the churches of his day to offer hope and instruction. In a letter to the church in Corinth, he declares,

> *We were under great pressure, far beyond our ability to endure, so that we despaired even of life. Indeed, in our hearts we felt the sentence of death. But this happened that we might not rely on ourselves but on God, who raises the dead. He has delivered us from such a deadly peril, and he will deliver us. On him we have set our hope that he will continue to deliver us.*
>
> — 2 Corinthians 1:8b – 10

You have the power, through God, to survive your circumstances; it is the same power given to Jesus through his most difficult time — his suffering on a cross. It sounds cliché, but in order to make the most of the environment and circumstances God has ordained for us, we have to rely on him.

Relying on ourselves will only cause us unnecessary pain and mess up potentially divinely appointed experiences for those with whom we come into contact. I think we all can agree that it is wise to trust God's sovereignty and continue to place our hope in him to work in us through our circumstances.

Second Opinion

Mike Foster, founder of People of the Second Chance

A. M. M.: You spend a lot of time around pastors and church leaders. In general, how do you perceive the overall health of leaders today?

M. F.: I think the perception is that at first glance pastors and church leaders are doing well. They are really skilled at saying the right things and managing image. But as soon as they open up just a bit about their struggle, you realize that there is a lot of pain, depression, hopelessness, and junk. The healthiest leaders I know are the ones who are transparent in their conversations with me and honest with the issues they struggle with. And the reverse is true also. The sickest leaders I know are the ones who are hyperperfect and obsessed with pleasing onlookers.

A. M. M.: Why do you think it's important for leaders to take care of themselves?

M. F.: It's the only way to have long-term success. Period. If you don't take care of yourself, you won't finish well. I've known too many Christian leaders who managed churches, ministries, staffs, and volunteers extremely well, yet they could not manage themselves. And that is what sank them. I truly believe that if you are intentional and strategic about taking care of yourself, everything else will fall into place.

A. M. M.: In your book *Deadly Viper Character Assassins*, you talk about seven assassins that can take leaders out when their guards are down. What are they?

M. F.: *The Assassin of Character Creep.* This stealth assassin is all about undermining our long-term success. Often a lifetime of work can be greatly affected by a few quick, careless decisions. Leaders often engage in "character creep" as they subtly and slowly cross lines.

The Assassin of Zi Qi Qi Ren. This assassin gets its name from a Chinese term meaning "self-deception while deceiving others." Subtly we can begin to shade the truth, refuse to face reality, and deceive ourselves. A leader begins to live with lies and travels down a slippery slope until this assassin takes him or her out.

The Assassin of Amped Emotions. Whether it's anger, jealousy, or amped-up horniness, our emotions can undermine our long-term success.

The Assassin of the Headless Sprinting Chicken. This assassin is all about maxed-out schedules and the lack of Sabbath in our lives.

The Assassin of Boom Chicka Wah Wah. One word: Sex.

The Bling Bling Assassin. This assassin makes us think we are defined by our stuff and leads us to be caught up in consumerism and a materialistic focus.

The High and Mighty Assassin. Leaders often do what they do in an unhealthy pursuit of proving their worth. Ego reveals itself in a devaluing of others to inflate oneself or in believing one's own press reports. The long-term effect of this behavior is a life that comes up short and is ultimately meaningless.

A. M. M.: When you start feeling stressed and burned-out, what are some things you notice?

M. F.: My biggest indicator of burnout is how I treat people. Because relationships mean so much to me and are such a core of my life, if I'm stressing or burning out, this is what is impacted. If I find myself losing my patience with people quickly and my thoughts become negative toward friends and family, or I find myself withdrawing from relationships, this means I've entered a danger zone.

What's most unfortunate, and probably not a unique situation, is that I take out my stress on the people I love the most. My wife and kids have been the clear victims of my not managing my life well. That's why I've become so diligent in addressing my physical, relational, emotional, and spiritual health.

Chapter 6: The Symptoms

Are you ready? Now is the time we have to be honest with ourselves.

Remember the tantrums you would throw when you were a little kid? This is where it gets easy to focus on the negative and to make the situation worse than it actually is.

On the other hand, denial is also an enemy of the truth. We can be so wrapped up in doing — or feeling that we have to do — that we are afraid to face the truth that we're on a brutal downward spiral into becoming completely ineffective for the kingdom.

In this chapter, we're going to take a look at the symptoms of burnout. Most of us have probably experienced these symptoms at some point in our lives, and just because we exhibit some of these signs doesn't necessarily mean we're burned-out. And there may be symptoms unique to you that aren't on this list.

The key is honest evaluation. I think it's wise to ask for outside opinions to assist you in developing a well-rounded snapshot of yourself. If you're wondering why you're behaving in a certain way, ask your spouse, your children, or the people closest to you to provide trustworthy insight.

Burnout versus Stress

Sometimes we have really stressful days. And sometimes those days turn into weeks. Seasons of stress come and go.

Burnout, however, is the result of cumulative stress developed over time. Dr. Archibald Hart, founder of the Hart Institute, describes how the symptoms of stress can turn into symptoms of burnout over the passage of time.[1]

Stress	Burnout
Stress is characterized by over engagement.	Burnout is a defense - characterized by disengagement.
The exhaustion of stress affects physical energy.	The exhaustion of burnout affects motivation and drive.
Stress produces disintegration.	Burnout produces demoralization.
Stress can best be understood as a loss of fuel and energy.	Burnout can best be understood as a loss of ideals and hope.
The depression of stress is produced by the body's need to protect itself and conserve energy.	The depression of burnout is caused by the grief engendered by the loss of ideals and hope.
Stress produces a sense of urgency and hyperactivity.	Burnout produces a sense of helplessness and hopelessness.

As you can see, symptoms of stress alone are fairly traumatic. As these persist without appropriate release, they worsen into burnout.

On the next few pages, I've provided checklists to help you identify some things you may be experiencing. As you work through these lists and note both the symptoms and how long you've been experiencing them, you should get a clear picture of your overall health in the four areas we've been discussing. Feel free to add other symptoms that may not be listed.

Spiritual Health

Check if you have symptom	Symptom	Duration (in months)
	No desire for Bible reading	
	No desire for prayer	
	Don't give cheerfully or sacrificially	
	Find yourself avoiding truth	
	Feel spiritually empty	
	Avoid accountable relationships	
	Lying (including little white lies)	
	Stealing (even in "small" ways)	

Check if you have symptom	Symptom	Duration (in months)

Physical Health

Check if you have symptom	Symptom	Duration (in months)
	Feeling tired all the time	
	Constant headaches	
	Consistent gastrointestinal issues	
	Weight gain or loss (how much?)	

	Carrying extra weight around midsection	
	Insomnia	
	Chest tightness / shortness of breath	
	Muscle aches / weakness	
	Pain in wrists or jaw (may indicate clenching hands or teeth in sleep)	
	Sighing frequently	
	Muscle twitches	

Emotional Health

Check if you have symptom	Symptom	Duration (in months)
	Easily angered / enraged	
	Snapping at small incidents	
	Negativity	
	Cynicism	
	Feeling as though you're the target ("everyone is out to get me")	
	Suspiciousness	
	Helplessness	
	Impulsiveness	
	Feeling sad	

	Lack of self-worth	
	Feeling empty	
	Don't feel satisfaction from achievements	
	Anxiety / worry	
	Panic attacks	
	Feeling as though you're on the verge of a breakdown	
	Using escapes such as alcohol, drugs, sex, TV, movies, or pornography	

Relational Health

Check if you have symptom	Symptom	Duration (in months)
	Withdraw from family and friends	
	Lose interest in spouse	
	Avoid children	
	Crave isolation / seclusion	
	Become anxious in social situations	
	Fear intimacy ("if they knew the real me, they wouldn't like me")	
	Find no joy in relationships	
	Dread going into work / participating in service	

Ok, So Now What?

I don't want to oversimplify things, but let's look back at your answers. Did you end up checking a lot of boxes? Have you been struggling with some of these issues for a while? Were you going through them, feeling each one intensely, saying, "Oh, my gosh, this is so me!!!"? Did you feel conviction setting in? Were some of the symptoms tough to evaluate?

If these last few pages are covered in pen scribble, chances are, Yes — yes, you're either burned-out, or on the brink of burnout.

Even though there is no "one size fits all" Band-Aid for healing burnout, we'll talk in the next few chapters about a few things you can do to help set you on the right path, if you choose to work through them — and continue working through them over time.

If you went through these lists and found that you seldom experienced the symptoms or have been experiencing some of them for just a short amount of time, you're probably not burned-out in the truest sense of the word.

HOWEVER (and yes, that's a big however) . . .

You picked up this book for a reason. Something about the subject of burnout and ministry struck a chord with you. Maybe you haven't hit bottom yet, but you sense it's looming out there in the road ahead. Maybe you're beginning to experience these stress symptoms now, and you want to stop them now before they overtake you and Satan takes you down. The chapters ahead will help.

And finally, maybe you're not the one who's burned-out, but you care for someone who is. You could be the spouse of a pastor, the friend of a co-volunteer, or an observant staff member or volunteer who sees the culture around you taking out those alongside you. You have the ability to lead (regardless of your title or position), and you desperately want those in your care to stay healthy and productive for the kingdom.

If that's the case, the upcoming chapters can serve as a guide on how to form a healthy ministry environment and also on how to take care of yourself in the four areas of health.

Second Opinion

Wayne Cordeiro, senior pastor,

New Hope Christian Fellowship, Oahu, Hawaii

A. M. M.: What were the first signs you experienced that caught you off guard and made you realize you might be burning out?

W. C.: Things that once came easily came hard, such as problem solving, relationships, and preaching — they all became increasingly more difficult. I found myself getting irritable and impatient at the little things in life. I also experienced an inability to focus or make decisions on general questions.

A. M. M.: What did the process look like when you decided to seek help?

W. C.: I called a psychologist first and then a cardiologist. I thought I was having heart problems because my heart began skipping, and I was losing my breath. But it turned out that I was having anxiety attacks several times a day.

A. M. M.: Many leaders struggle with feeling that they can't take a break — fearing that if they do, something won't get done. If someone is burning out but feels that obligation, what advice would you give them?

W. C.: The first thing is to make the symptoms known to close confidants or a church board member you trust. But get help. The longer you ignore the issue and refuse to deal with it, the harder it is to detect. A diminishing of ministry capacity is next, and the longer the pattern remains, the harder it is to bounce back from the flatline. It took me three years to bounce back.

A. M. M.: What are some practices you've changed since your burnout?

W. C.: I don't wait till I'm fried before I take a break anymore. If you wait, it's too late. As they say in long-distance racing, "If you wait until you're thirsty before you drink water, you are already dehydrated." I also take more time to enjoy life. It is still a very difficult discipline for me since I intensely love what I do. I enjoy immensely using for God's glory the gifts that he gave me. However, an unguarded strength can become your greatest weakness. Unknowingly, the road to success and the road to a nervous breakdown became the same road.

Also, one of the best things I did was to identify those things in my life that are most important, and I invest in them each day. I run my life a bit more slowly these days, but I do it with far more traction. I have begun to strengthen my strengths as my new challenge rather than trying to prop up my weaknesses. I recognize them, but instead of driving myself to better those areas, I admit them, get others to help, and stay in my strengths. The last thing is I've learned that God has made me to be a leader, not a "manager." I was pulled in to "managing" for a few years as my main course. That diminished my leadership immune system, and I became susceptible to contagious maladies such as discouragement, exasperation, and being demotivated by others. Leaders don't catch passing emotional illnesses often, but when we are burned-out, we do. Then we isolate ourselves to keep from being affected.

PART 3

GETTING BETTER: SIX PRINCIPLES FOR RECOVERY

Some of the things I'm going to say in the rest of this book may not sit well with your comfort zone. Not to sound sadistic, but it is my sincere hope that the questions and challenges that are to come are a little painful.

Sometimes in order to heal, we have to hurt first. If you've ever dislocated your shoulder, you know this. Someone has to take hold of your arm and shove it back into its socket. It hurts like fire. But if you let your arm stay out of its socket, it wouldn't do you a lick of good, now, would it?

If you're not ready to make some serious changes in your life right now, may I suggest you put this book down? I know I sometimes read books just to read them — I don't make any real effort to make changes in my life.

Please don't do that.

If you're content to live a completely unfulfilled life, dreading each day, feeling miserable, and, worst of all, not living the life God has given you and intended for you, go ahead and close up shop and continue wasting away. I really wish you the best, but you've got to be ready and committed to make serious changes — and make them right now.

If you're ready to change — if you know you can't go on living in the state you're in, with your joy completely stolen and your life being destroyed — let's continue, shall we?

Remember, there is no magic pill to help you. Chances are none of this material will be new to you. But as you commit to getting very real with a very real God and to living an abundant life, these next steps will help you begin the journey to recovery.

There are many other practical steps we'll discuss later, but I truly believe that reflecting on and taking in these six principles will provide a great foundation for making practical decisions in the future. After we become familiar with each of the steps, we'll apply them to the four individual areas of health in subsequent chapters.

Chapter 7: Principle 1
Reconnect with your Savior

"The thief comes only to steal and kill and destroy; I have come that they may have life, and have it to the full."

— John 10:10

When I considered adding some new material to the first edition of Mad Church Disease, I reached out to a few trusted pastors I knew who read it for feedback. One of the most thoughtful responses came from my friend Ryan, a pastor in Holland, Michigan.

He said,

"What is the Gospel for the burned out or near burned out? To get to a point where you are burned out or near it you have been trusting something other than God for some time."

Zing. Ryan hit the nail on the head. His comment made me want to press delete on most of my work and start a whole new book. I read over what I wrote the first time around and agree – although there's a lot of practical insight in this book, there's also a lot of "doing" and not a lot of challenge to "be."

I wondered, "How do I balance providing practical help that has given so many people a good jumping-off point with something that's not tangible?" After toying around with several options, I decided that the first "Recovery Principle" simply needed to be on being.

I could write an entirely new book on this idea, but I know this book's job is to be practical and broad. So, I thought the best place to talk about "just being" was before you got to any of the "doing."

Before you change your eating habits, sign up for yoga, cut your hours back and join a small group, take a deep breath.

We look for instant fixes. We feel empty, and we want to feel full. God promised us fullness, right? Why don't we sense that completeness? We search for whatever we think will tide us over.

And what we do find is only a cheap fix. It's not what God intended.

The Greek word perissos is translated "full" in John 10:10. It doesn't mean happy. It doesn't mean comfortable. It doesn't mean prosperous or wealthy.

Perissos means "in abundance."

Overflowing.

Life overflowing.

Not a long life, or even a healthy one. The life in John 10:10 is the life that was made possible, brought into existence, so to speak, when Jesus sacrificed for us. It's eternal life. And the Greek word for "life" (zom en) implies a life that is present now and in the future.

"I have come" (the work is already done) . . .

"That they may have"

(there's nothing you can do to earn it — so just accept it) . . .

"Life."

We need to realize that the abundant life God has for you already exists!

It's ours.

We need to rest in that fact.

And I mean really rest.

But What about Sacrifice?

Ministry does require sacrifice. The Christian life requires sacrifice. In his letter to the Romans, Paul writes,

> I urge you, brothers, in view of God's mercy, to offer your bodies as living sacrifices, holy and pleasing to God — this is your spiritual act of worship.
> — Romans 12:1

When Jesus died on the cross, the need for Old Testament sacrifices died with him. Jesus is and was and always will be the ultimate sacrifice.

God's grace is amazing, and it is beyond my understanding how and why he continues to use us in spite of our frailties. Yet my heart breaks because I believe the church (the church universal) is not doing all we can do. We are not completely offering our individual lives as holy and living sacrifices.

God has always wanted sacrifices that come from humble hearts that look to him in faith, hearts infused with the new life of the Holy Spirit, hearts transformed to live and love like Jesus. He does not want the sacrifices of those who do not live holy and pleasing lives. The Old Testament prophets make it clear that God would prefer that people don't worship him at all than that they worship him while living a lifestyle of injustice (see Isaiah 1:11 – 17; Amos 5:21 – 24; Malachi 1:10 – 11).

How can we truly offer ourselves as the living sacrifices God requires?

Realize there's a difference between what you feel you must sacrifice and what God actually requires.

The only sacrifice he requires is you.

You to him.

We are living sacrifices, holy and pleasing to God.

Offering ourselves up to him is our act of worship.

And that is the only sacrifice he requires.

Live and rest fully and abundantly in that promise. His mercy and his grace will take care of the rest.

Sabbath

Many books have been written on the importance of the Sabbath. Countless leadership talks have encouraged us to take appropriate rest. We talk about it, pray about it, and even say we're going to do it — but for the most part, we don't change a thing!

When we think of Sabbath, we think of resting on the seventh day. After all, God took six days to create the world. On the seventh day, he rested. We might think of Sabbath as a reward for our hard work.

However, let me challenge you to think of Sabbath in a different way.

First, we need to recognize that God didn't need to rest. He is God. But he rested anyway. He created human beings with a need for a day in which they could step aside from the busyness and the mundane in order to refocus and be restored. God created all things, and then took a day of rest, knowing he was setting the ultimate example.

In *Sit, Walk, Stand*, Watchman Nee describes the Sabbath:

> *Where did [Adam] stand in relation to that rest of God? Adam, we are told, was created on the sixth day. Clearly, then, he had no part in those first six days of work, for he came into being only at their end. God's seventh day was, in fact, Adam's first. Where God worked six days and then enjoyed his Sabbath rest, Adam began his life with the Sabbath; for God works before he rests, while man must first enter into God's rest, and then alone can he work.[3]*

The New Testament often uses the word rest to describe the good news of grace and salvation proclaimed in Jesus Christ (see, for example, Matthew 11:28; Hebrews 4:2 – 3).[4] So the Sabbath doesn't just signify a day of rest but defines why we are able to rest, and should rest, because of the connection to the gospel. Salvation itself begins in rest — knowing that Jesus has already accomplished perfection in his life and death. We can only truly rest by realizing we have been made complete in Jesus Christ. The Sabbath isn't only referring to one particular day in the seven days of the week. It also points to our entering into God's eternal rest, where kingdom work has already been accomplished.

Watchman Nee continues:

> *And here is the gospel: that God has gone one stage further and has completed also the work of redemption, and that we need to do nothing whatever to merit it, but can enter by faith directly into the values of his finished work.*[5]

If you think that wanting to keep busy all the time is a product of -modern-day technology, take a look at what the prophet Isaiah declared:

This is what the Sovereign LORD, the Holy One of Israel, says:

"In repentance and rest is your salvation,
>   in quietness and trust is your strength,
>   but you would have none of it."

                                                            — Isaiah 30:15

Even thousands of years ago, mankind refused the beautiful gift of rest. Why do we always prefer the opposite? In fact, please allow me the liberty of flipping this verse into its opposite form.

"In rebellion and work is your demise,
>   in noisiness and distrust is your weakness,
>   and you will have it all the time."

Why do those words ring so true?

Because we are believing lies!

We believe lies that tell us that our worth is in our productivity. We believe lies that say you can't trust anybody with your problems. We are so tempted by the glitz and glamour of sacrifice and doing things for Christ that we ignore the work Christ has already done in us. We allow false humility and large egos to drive us into eighty-hour weeks and an unholy commitment to self-reliance.

And when we are relying on ourselves, we aren't relying on God.

Self-reliance quietly whispers to our souls, "You don't need rest. You don't need to refresh. You can do everything on your own. God is helping you, right?"

In Mark 6, Jesus sends the apostles out two by two to do his work. It was one of those "all hands on deck" kind of seasons. They were incredibly busy, incredibly hurried. And even as they filed their report with Jesus, there was such a hustle and bustle of activity around them that they didn't have a chance to eat.

Busy? Hurried? Skipping meals?

Yep. Sounds like ministry.

And they pushed through.

After spending some time with Jesus, instead of heading straight back into their ministry, they are commanded to rest.

"Come with me by yourselves to a quiet place and get some rest" (Mark 6:31).

Jesus knew that the apostles needed to rest.

> Alone.

> But at the same time — with him.

Jesus is telling you to come to him to find rest. You don't need a burning bush. He tells you through Scripture. He tells you through circumstances and people. He speaks this invitation to you when your soul is empty and your heart can't take anymore.

You need rest. Rest in knowing that the work has already been done on a cross. Your only work is to accept it and listen to the sweet words of Christ lavishing his love over you.

Chapter 8: Principle 2
Accept Responsibility for Your Decisions

I was seven years old. My parents had just become owners of their first "newish" car — a 1985 Dodge Ramcharger in a beautiful midnight-blue. And with my allowance, I had just purchased a shiny metal hair clip. As I was waiting for my parents to leave church one evening, I popped the clip out of my hair and started doodling in that beautiful midnight-blue paint. I realized my clip was pretty sharp and thought I'd try to write my name underneath the door handle. Slowly I carved the letters A-N-N-E-M-A-R-I-E on the door. Before I finished dotting my "I," a friend came over and asked if I wanted to play. I ran off with her, leaving the freshly vandalized door far from my thoughts.

A little while later at home, I was minding my own business in my room. My dad came storming in, livid. He asked if I had written my name on the car.

"No," I confidently said.

He kept asking. I kept denying.

Finally, he looked down to see what I was playing with. It was a Care Bears tape recorder.

Without a second thought, he snatched it off the floor, threw it back down, and with his big size-10 shoes, stepped on it. No, stomped on it. Over and over and over again. Until all that was left were springs and broken pieces of plastic scattered on the floor.

I was stunned. I was angry. I was sad.

I began bawling.

He looked at me, still upset, and said, "If you would've just owned up to what you did, you wouldn't be crying right now," and left my room.

. . .

There may be many external reasons why you're burned-out. Your senior pastor could be a jerk. You may have had some difficult health issues, and now you're just trying to make ends meet because of all the medical bills that have piled up. Maybe you have a chemical imbalance and struggle with depression.

However, we all make choices. And the effect of the decisions you have made over time has led you now to burnout.

I'm going to say that again.

The effect of the decisions you have made over time has led you now to burnout.

That may be a tough pill to swallow. But please, let it soak in a little bit. The first step in overcoming burnout is to own up to the decisions that have led you here.

No human is perfect. However, we do have the exact same Spirit Jesus had guiding him. The one man who endured more pain and suffering than any other man in the course of history. He definitely exhibited symptoms of stress. Sleepless nights. Desperate cries to the Father. Great temptations. Unbelievably harsh external circumstances. Yet because of his decisions, his resilience through thirty-three years of life was unbreakable.

You are responsible for the decisions you have made. The late nights. The double cheeseburgers. The neglect of your Bible, your prayer time, your family. Those were your decisions.

The first step on this path is taking responsibility. You are responsible both for the choices you've made in life and for seeking God's plan for your healing. Are you ready?

Healing from Abuse

There is one exception to this rule of taking ownership — and a group of people whom I need to address. If you were abused — physically, sexually, spiritually or emotionally — at some point in your life, you had no choice in that decision, even though the circumstances still affect you greatly today and can even contribute to burnout.

Somebody hurt you, and regardless of the role you believed you played in that abuse, you cannot accept responsibility for your abuser's actions.

I understand the long-term effect this has on you, and I'm here to offer you some hope before we move on. Even though you have no way of changing the past or changing what happened to you, even though you were in no way responsible for what happened, you can choose how to handle the fallout that inevitably occurs.

For a brief time in high school, someone I trusted sexually abused me. For the first few years after it happened, I medicated the hurt in a variety of unhealthy ways. The next few years, I simply blunted my emotions so I didn't have to feel anything at all. Maybe you can relate.

Recently, I met a wise and godly woman. She was my counselor, and she helped me realize that, even though I needed to let go of the guilt I was carrying in thinking that the abuse was my fault; I also needed to take responsibility for working through the pain.

It was irresponsible to cover up the hurt or ignore it. God had so much more waiting for me if only I could face the pain and the loss, grieve it, and then begin to accept the good he had planned.

This isn't me saying, "Just get over it." In the same way, I urge you, desperately urge you, to take responsibility for your recovery from the abuse — no matter whether you were abused as a child or even as an adult. The truth is, abuse can occur anywhere and any time in ministry.

Accept the pain and loss and ask God to show you what he has planned for your healing. I promise he will do more in your mind and heart than you can ever ask or imagine.

Rx:

Identify specific decisions you have made that have set you up as an easy target for Satan to take down.

List some barriers to your becoming fully restored. Some examples to get you started are denial, fear of failure, and so on.

What are some steps you can take within the next week to begin accepting responsibility for your past decisions? Is there someone you need to confess or apologize to?

Chapter 9: Principle 3
Change Your Purpose

On a stretch of highway leading to my parents' house are a series of billboards. Most of them spell out a word in giant red letters.

REPENT!!!

The word repent has developed an evangelical extremist stigma over the last forty years. I'm reminded of the incoherent man roaming around downtown wearing a sandwich board, screaming poorly memorized, out-of-context verses from the book of Revelation. Or I think of "repenting" from listening to "the devil's music" when I was in high school, which also led me to throw out all my country music CDs. (Notice I threw out just the country ones. Snoop Dog stayed.)

Sometimes we do need a big billboard and giant red letters to get our attention. We need the extreme.

REPENT!!!

Repent comes from the Greek word metanoeam which literally means, "to change one's mind or purpose."[1]

Let's face it: If we're not experiencing the abundant life described in John 10:10, we've gotten off course somewhere. We need to change our mind. We need to change our purpose.

Webster's Collegiate Dictionary defines purpose as "something to be set up as an object or end to be attained: intention, resolution, determination."

If you're burned-out, whatever it is you're trying to attain needs to be changed.

So, what is it?

Are you trying to run the best children's ministry in the country? Are you attempting to grow your church by two hundred people this year? Are you trying to make your church's print pieces the slickest in town? Have the most amazing worship service? Earn your fifth master's degree?

All of the above are extremely noble and worthy causes. You can be passionate about these things. You can run hard after them. You can do them with excellence.

But if these things are your purpose, I hate to tell you this, but you're chasing after the wrong thing. Change the message you hear. These things are your *calling*. They are not your purpose.

If you take God's call on your life and turn it into your purpose in life, you will burn out.

Don't believe me?

Go back to the chapter on symptoms and revisit those items you checked off. Are you burned out? Or almost burned out? The only way to get back on track is to change your purpose.

What is Our Purpose?

The gospel writer Mark records for us God's greatest command:

> *"The most important [commandment]," answered Jesus, "is this: 'Hear, O Israel, the Lord our God, the Lord is one. Love the Lord your God with all your heart and with all your soul and with all your mind and with all your strength.' The second is this: 'Love your neighbor as yourself.' There is no commandment greater than these."*
>
> — Mark 12:29 – 31

It doesn't say, "The greatest commandment is to love your job with all your heart, soul, mind, and strength."

It doesn't say, "The greatest commandment is to love your calling with all your heart, soul, mind, and strength."

It doesn't even say, "Love the church with all your heart, soul, mind, and strength."

The greatest commandment.

Love the Lord your God.

With all your heart.

With all your soul.

With all your mind.

With all your strength.

And next?

Love your neighbor as yourself.

Isn't it interesting how the four areas of health we are measuring are the same areas of health God commands us to love him with, so we in turn can show our neighbors the life-changing love of Christ?

God promises us life if we obey his commands. He clearly wants to give us life. An abundant life.

If you are burned-out . . .

If you haven't been seeking God's true purpose for your life . . .

If you need to change your course and love God with all your heart, soul, mind, and strength . . .

Now is the time.

Stop what you've been doing — what you've always been doing — and turn around.

Change your purpose.

There's no better time than right now.

Rx:

If you're burned-out, take a look at why. What is it that you have been chasing? Even with the best intentions, if we aren't committed to pursuing a loving relationship with our Creator, we are destined to fail. What are the things you are loving with all your heart, soul, mind, and strength?

What steps can you take this week to begin changing your course?

Chapter 10: Principle 4
Make a Plan

In the next couple of chapters, we'll talk about practical ways to begin making changes in order to prevent burnout or to begin the journey of healing from burnout. It's very important that you make plans to change and commit to follow through with these plans. Good intentions are great. But they won't take you anywhere. Solomon shares insight on the importance of making plans:

> A wicked man puts up a bold front,
>> but an upright man gives thought to his ways.
>
> — Proverbs 21:29

Our good intentions are just that — a bold front. Our plans may sound impressive, but they're nothing but a facade unless we put intention and action to them.

When making plans, it's easy to get overwhelmed. Patience is absolutely essential. There seems to be so much we need to work on and "fix" that it will be easy to become discouraged. It's OK to start slowly. Small steps over time can make a big difference — and not only that, God will honor your obedience in ways beyond what we can humanly accomplish. As we make plans, we should do so with God's purpose in mind. We should seek his vision for our lives. Wise Solomon writes,

> In his heart a man plans his course, but the LORD determines his steps.
>
> — Proverbs 16:9

Ask God to show you the decisions you need to make first. What steps are most important for you to take right now? He'll be faithful in showing you.

As the Bible teaches,

> Commit to the LORD whatever you do,
>> and your plans will succeed.
>
> — Proverbs 16:3

When it comes to making plans that will succeed, you must commit them to the Lord. It also doesn't hurt to write them down and commit them to yourself.

By putting pen to paper (or fingers to keyboard), you're taking your thoughts and good intentions and putting them into a tangible form. By seeing your goals spelled out, you're more likely to follow through with them. There's something about the written word that subconsciously implies commitment.

And when you commit those plans to God, if they're in line with his will, they'll succeed. It's a promise.

Rx:

This is where the rubber meets the road. You've owned up to your decisions that have taken you down the path to burnout. You've identified your course in life and have decided to get back on the right road. Now it's time to make some definitive plans. In the next four chapters, you'll be asked to make specific plans for the four areas of health. It is vitally important that you humbly seek God in prayer as you make these plans and that you commit to them by writing them down.

In the space below, ask God to begin revealing his plans for you. Jot down some initial impressions as you seek God's will. Ask him for the strength you'll need to make tough choices and to commit to whatever it is he shows you.

Chapter 11: Principle 5
Create Boundaries

We want to be all things to all people. Accessible. Helpful. Always available to listen. When we're not, we think we're being selfish. What if we don't love someone the way Jesus would love someone?

Would Jesus ever say no to people?

Yes.

In Luke's gospel, we learn that Jesus spends quite a bit of time in a town called Capernaum. He heals the sick. He drives out demons. He truly exerts his authority over intense spiritual powers and shows compassion in the midst of evil. Because of this, news of his ability travels fast and far.

At the end of Luke 4, Jesus retreats. He needs to rest. He knows it's time to move on to other cities. But the people find him. They crowd him and beg him to stay.

Much more healing needs to take place. Many other people need his touch.

His response?

No.

"I must preach the good news of the kingdom of God to the other towns also, because that is why I was sent" (Luke 4:43).

Jesus wasn't sent to heal people in just one small corner of the world. He was sent to heal the world. If Jesus failed to establish boundaries but devoted himself instead to the things right in front of him, the rest of the world would suffer.

In the same way, we have to look at the entire kingdom picture when we review our to-do lists. When we see the people we "need" to talk to, the events we "must" plan, the emails that "have to be" answered . . .

We must ask ourselves. . .

Really?

Creating boundaries isn't selfish. It's necessary.

Craig Groeschel, senior pastor of LifeChurch.tv, sets a pretty amazing example when it comes to setting boundaries for his evenings. When I asked him what boundaries he had in place to protect that, he responded,

> *I'm away from home one night a week — that's when I'm preaching on Saturday nights. We are literally together six nights a week as a family. The key to developing that environment is protecting our time in the evenings. I don't do evening meetings, don't schedule dinner meetings, and don't have the elders meeting in the evening. We have those meetings early in the morning or at lunchtime. I get home around 5:15 every night, and that is practically set in stone. You should design your ministry around your family values. It can be challenging because not every staff person can do that all the time, but you can to some degree.*

When we create boundaries, we aren't saying to the world, "I can't help you." Instead, we're saying, "I must focus intentionally on the specific things God has placed right now in my direct influence." By saying no to people and to things that are not contained within God's distinct vision for our lives, we're actually saying yes to his sovereignty. He knows the best way for his will to be accomplished. For us to assume we can handle more is rebellious and counterproductive.

Rx

In order to heal, you will have to create boundaries in all areas of your health. At first, expect it to be difficult when you start using one of the most important words in your healing — "NO!" You may feel guilty for saying it. People may get angry at you for saying it. But you must say it!

List three to five areas in which you know boundaries will be difficult to create and maintain. These can be about how you spend your time or how you can make changes in your relationships or in areas in ministry you know need adjustment.

1.

2.

3.

4.

5.

Write a prayer asking God to help you understand the importance of setting boundaries and to begin giving you the courage you will need to establish and follow through on them.

Chapter 12: Principle 6
Find ~~Accountability~~ Authentic Relationships

In the first edition of this book, this chapter was titled "Find Accountability." Maybe it's just my love of words, but I can't stand what the word "accountability" has become in the last 10 years. The original meaning of it, being willing to take responsibility, has changed in our church circles to "let me give you a report of what I did wrong and right this week and let me hear yours and we'll meet again next week to check back." Rarely is there any movement – it becomes a behavioral check-in system.

After writing my book *Lean on Me* (October 2014), I made a meaningful shift in the way I look at accountability and I adapted the term "Accountability Partner" to "Authenticity Partner." Instead of having a relationship based on protocol, having an Authenticity Partner is about allowing someone to have access to the truest part of who you are. They have permission to ask the difficult questions and to follow Biblical reproach when necessary. They are committed to *you*, not to your meeting. You, in essence, surrender a part of your freedom over to them. I write about this extensively in *Lean on Me* if it's something that interests you.

When I first wrote this book, I was forever stuck in writing this section. I recently moved, and with the move, my biweekly lunch with my Authenticity Partner disappeared. To not be in an accountable relationship is completely unacceptable. And you can only go so long playing the "I don't know anyone" card.

So how could I write a section about accountability without having that relationship in my own life? The answer? I couldn't. For a week I stared at this page and attempted to dream up ways to convey the importance of an authentic relationship, but God put a providential writer's block in my path.

Trust takes time. Relationships take time. And as I spend more time getting to know people in my new town, I was sure relationships would naturally develop and I'd be able to share those very personal things with someone face-to-face. But until that happened, I couldn't wait.

I emailed a friend of mine who lives in Alabama. We've known each other for a couple of years and have shared similar struggles both personally and in ministry. Also, we're both married, and we both work in a church. And most important, I trust her. I can share my darkest struggles with her. I proceeded to set up a regular time to chat about specific things we were dealing with.

Over time, I developed friendships. In fact, over the last four years of my life, those relationships have been truly life saving. (Not to beat a dead horse or sell you something, but if you find close relationships tough to navigate, *Lean on Me* may be a valuable resource for you). It takes intentionality and vulnerability, but we all need people we can trust, and who can trust us back.

When you begin the process of healing from burnout, you're going to uncover some ugly things about yourself. And you're going to want to hide these ugly things under a big rock.

That won't do you any good, now, will it?

Let's think of things that thrive in dark places:

Mold

> Mildew

> > Germs

> > > Rats

> > > > Smelly, gross things

Nothing really good.

The Bible is clear: Darkness and light cannot coexist.

If we keep things in the dark, we'll never be completely free of them.

Not only are authentic relationships important for areas of weakness in our lives;

they're also necessary for the areas in which God is growing us.

As you work through the next chapters that deal with each area of health, you'll be asked to set goals for yourself in every area. After you set milestones, and even after you write them down, another way to show your commitment to change is by sharing these goals with another person who will ask the hard question: Are you making progress on what you said you would do?

Rx

We need accountability *and* authenticity in our lives. We need people to pray for us as we struggle and as we grow. As you prepare to make some long-term, life-changing decisions, identify those layers of accountability *and* authenticity you need to have in your life.

In the space below, make a list of those people you feel comfortable asking to help you in the process of recovering from burnout. If you aren't in any authentic relationships, write a prayer asking God to bring to your mind people you should consider. He'll be faithful in showing you — because community is in his plan for your life!

PART 4

PRACTICAL STEPS FOR HEALTHY MINISTRY

I know I've said this before, but there are no magic pills that will help you go from burned-out and ready to throw in the towel to the most energetic and positive person in the world. We're going to discuss some practical ways to make your life healthier overall. However, I need you to keep in mind a couple of things:

- Not all of these will apply to everyone.

- This is a place to get you started. Once you're done reading, if you stop growing, you'll likely revert to old habits.

After reading many stories and realizing the breadth of how burnout affects everyone uniquely, I had to choose the greatest common denominators. Burnout hits people in all roles and abilities, and because of the broad spectrum, I can't cover every symptom or cause out there.

You are going to be contributing to these chapters as much, if not more, than I have. You'll have room to write and sort through plans for all of the areas of health. This should give you a solid platform for making some life-changing decisions. Remember — in the end, this change is up to you!

Everyone's journey is unique, and I am praying that as you work through issues in each of these areas, God will speak to you and reveal himself in amazing ways.

Chapter 13: Spiritual Health

Everybody thinks of changing humanity and nobody thinks of changing himself.

— Leo Tolstoy

Becoming spiritually healthy should be your primary focus in your recovery from burnout. Without this element, you can be physically fit, relationally graceful, and emotionally sturdy, but you will still be limiting the Holy Spirit's ability to work in your life.

Right now, you may be spiritually empty and dry. Your sensitivity to the sin in your own life has diminished. You know you're not in regular fellowship with God, and right now you don't even care. Well, you might feel like you don't care, but the fact that you are reading this book is telling me otherwise.

As leaders, we are charged with the care of those God has entrusted to us. Without a high spiritual intake, our spiritual output will be low — if it exists at all. Unfortunately, because many of us are suffering spiritually, our churches and communities are suffering spiritually too.

The Bible outlines many spiritual disciplines that are essential to a believer's spiritual health. Neglecting one or more of the spiritual disciplines is probably the best way to put our spiritual health on a downward spiral. Here are five disciplines that have been vital ingredients in my own spiritual health.

Prayer

Key Scriptures

And pray in the Spirit on all occasions with all kinds of prayers and requests. With this in mind, be alert and always keep on praying for all the saints.

— Ephesians 6:18

Do not be anxious about anything, but in everything, by prayer and petition, with thanksgiving, present your requests to God.

— Philippians 4:6

Be joyful always; pray continually; give thanks in all circumstances, for this is God's will for you in Christ Jesus.

— 1 Thessalonians 5:16 – 18

Before my trip to Africa, I never spent a significant time away from a close friend or family member. Even though my parents live across the country from me, I have (a minimum) of a weekly phone chat with my mom. Sometimes it's more, and there's always various social media to keep up with on mundane life.

However, I knew that when I was in Africa, I wouldn't be able to talk on the phone. And I honestly can't remember one time my mom and I have gone more than a week without talking to each other.

After being in Africa for several days, I realized that I missed talking to her. Not only because I love her, but also because she understands me so intimately. I don't even have to use words sometimes for her to know what I'm thinking or feeling. She can see something in my demeanor or hear something in my voice that clues her in on what I'm going through.

Even though I was able to talk to the people who were with me on the trip, it was still difficult to process with them everything I was experiencing because, for the most part, we came into the trip as total strangers. They didn't know me as intimately as my mom does. Plus, she was a missionary to Venezuela in her twenties. Not being able to share even the smallest things with her on this trip caused me to shut down inside. I wasn't able to process everything completely.

God knows us even more intimately than our families do. And he designed us to express our deepest thoughts and longings to him. The Bible says we don't even have to use words.

When we break away from prayer, whether we consciously realize it or not, we're also breaking away from our natural design to talk and listen to our Creator. And without that line of communication flowing in both directions, we'll begin to burn out.

Meditation and Study of Scripture

Key Scriptures

> Do not let this Book of the Law depart from your mouth; meditate on it day and night, so that you may be careful to do everything written in it. Then you will be prosperous and successful.
>
> — Joshua 1:8

> I remember the days of long ago;
>
> > I meditate on all your works
> > and consider what your hands have done.
>
> — Psalm 143:5

Studying Scripture is fundamental to our spiritual health. The Bible is God's words and instructions to us. The Holy Spirit illuminates Scripture to us. We are taught about God's character. We are reminded of God's faithfulness in the past. We are instructed on how to live holy lives of love. We are convicted through Scripture. During the times when I'm faithful, I find it hard to explain how Scripture overflows from my mind and my heart and is applied constantly throughout my day. I have personally struggled with consistent Bible study. My life seems to get too busy, and I honestly sometimes just blow it off because I'm running around "doing things for God." And during the seasons when I am lazy and neglect time in God's Word, I realize how simple it is to justify sin in my life. I lose focus on truth.

Speaking of focus, Webster's Collegiate Dictionary defines meditate as "to focus one's thoughts on: reflect on or ponder over," and the Bible shares with us the importance of both Bible study and meditation. We typically think of meditation as something we do in solitude —

which it absolutely can be. And that particular kind of meditation is incredibly essential to our spiritual health too.

Even when we're not in solitude, we are all meditating on something. What is it that holds your attention all day long? The psalmist realizes that we are meditate by nature, and he directs us to the One who is the always appropriate object of our meditation:

I will sing to the LORD all my life;

I will sing praise to my God as long as I live.

May my meditation be pleasing to him,
as I rejoice in the LORD.

— Psalm 104:33 – 34

If our thoughts and hearts are focused on things outside of God's plan for us, we'll soon lose sight of his work in our lives and in the world around us.

Worship

Key Scriptures

"Yet a time is coming and has now come when the true worshipers will worship the Father in spirit and truth, for they are the kind of worshipers the Father seeks. God is spirit, and his worshipers must worship in spirit and in truth."

— John 4:23 – 24

Everyone was filled with awe, and many wonders and miraculous signs were done by the apostles. All the believers were together and had everything in common. Selling their possessions and goods, they gave to anyone as he had need. Every day they continued to meet together in the temple courts. They broke bread in their homes and ate together with glad and sincere hearts, praising God and enjoying the favor of all the people. And the Lord added to their number daily those who were being saved.

— Acts 2:43 – 47

Worship is another word we tend to misconstrue over time. It's become synonymous with music or a service on the weekend. So, let's just define worship in the context of a spiritual discipline as "expressing our dependence on the Holy Spirit by reflecting on and celebrating all of the things God has done for us and is to us." We do this both individually in our day-to-day living and corporately with other believers.

When you serve in ministry in any capacity, it's easy to become numb to the "emotion" we sometimes experience as we worship. It's easy to lose the awe Paul describes in Acts 2. And after we lose that awe, it's easy to become closed off or even cynical. Worship becomes nothing but an act, and when we go through the motions, we pull away from what God intended in John 4:23 – 24. We are no longer worshiping in spirit and in truth.

Service

Key Scripture

When he had finished washing their feet, he put on his clothes and returned to his place. "Do you understand what I have done for you?" he asked them. "You call me 'Teacher' and 'Lord,' and rightly so, for that is what I am. Now that I, your Lord and Teacher, have washed your feet, you also should wash one another's feet. I have set you an example that you should do as I have done for you. I tell you the truth, no servant is greater than his master, nor is a messenger greater than the one who sent him. Now that you know these things, you will be blessed if you do them."

— John 13:12 – 17

The greatest One of all washed the feet of his disciples — including the one who betrayed him. This story is the classic example of biblical service.

Of all the disciplines, it would seem natural that service would come easily. Many times, however, we confuse self-righteous service with true service.[1]

Self-righteous service	True service
Self-righteous service comes through human effort; it delights in plans and organizational charts.	True service comes from a relationship with Jesus Christ. Energy is expended, but it is not feverish.
Self-righteous service is impressed with the "big deal"; it is concerned with noteworthy outcomes.	True service does not distinguish big projects from small, and when the difference is noted, the small task is often found to be more important.
Self-righteous service requires external rewards; it needs to be appreciated (subject to appropriate "religious modesty," of course).	True service is content in hiddenness. It does not fear attention, but it does not seek it. The divine nod of approval is enough.
Self-righteous service is concerned with results. It avoids service if the outcome might fall below expectations.	True service does not need to see results; it delights only in the service. It can serve both enemies and the ungrateful.
Self-righteous service picks and chooses whom to serve.	True service is indiscriminate.

Self-righteous service	True service
Self-righteous service is affected by moods and whims; it exists only when there is a feeling to serve ("moved by the Spirit," as we say).	True service ministers simply and faithfully because there is a need.
Self-righteous service is temporary, mainly by way of occasional projects and "special" acts.	True service is a life-style.
Self-righteous service is insensitive. It forces itself in and demands the opportunity to help.	True service listens with tenderness and patience before acting.
Self-righteous service fractures community; once the religious trappings are removed, it focuses mainly on self-glorification.	True service builds community. It is caring and quiet and unpretentious.

Self-righteous service is service out of our own will and out of our own strength. We will burn out in no time. However, true service — the kind that is inspired by the Holy Spirit working in our lives — requires us to depend on God's strength.

Submission

Key Scriptures

> "Love the Lord your God with all your heart and with all your soul and with all your mind and with all your strength."
>
> — Mark 12:30

> Submit yourselves, then, to God. Resist the devil, and he will flee from you.
>
> — James 4:7

Submission is the enemy of our human will and the opposite of everything our hearts desire. We crave our rights. We demand our freedom.

Not our will, Lord, but yours be done. That should be our prayer.

It's interesting that in James 4:7 the biblical writer juxtaposes a sentence about submission with a sentence about the devil.

The tension between pursuing our own desires, hopes, and dreams and pursuing what God has for us can cause such confusion and distraction. And this is where Satan loves to get us every time.

The Greek word hypotassm ("submit") in James 4:7 has the sense of "lining up under another." Thinking of submission in a military context, we have the picture of soldiers coming under the authority of their officers. So too the apostle Paul instructs us to place ourselves in God's hands and to put on the full armor of God to be ready for spiritual warfare:

> Finally, be strong in the Lord and in his mighty power. Put on the full armor of God so that you can take your stand against the devil's schemes. For our struggle is not against flesh and blood, but against the rulers, against the authorities, against the powers of this dark world and against

the spiritual forces of evil in the heavenly realms.

— Ephesians 6:10 – 12

It's a spiritual uphill battle to live the abundant life God has called us to. John tells us in John 10:10 that the enemy's sole purpose — his only intent — is to destroy us. However, by equipping ourselves with the armor of God and by submitting to him (relying on his protection and his power), we are promised that the devil will flee.

And we are promised life to the full.

Respond

Principle 1: Reconnect with your Savior

Using the space below or in your own journal, write a prayer or a poem or draw something that helps you understand that God has taken care of you. That it may be in our nature to hide, but it's in his nature to pursue you. Especially in this chapter, spend some time meditating on Scripture, praying, journaling. Go for a walk. Do whatever it takes to get out of your head space and into the truth about what God thinks about you.

Principle 2: Own Up

1. Describe your approach to key spiritual disciplines over the last six months. Has it been constant and open? Or has it been lacking in both quality and quantity?
   - prayer
   - meditation and study of Scripture
   - worship
   - service
   - submission

2. What are some specific things you have done to contribute to the current state of your spiritual health?

3. Good or bad, do you accept your role in this? How?

Principle 3: Change Your Purpose

1. Sometimes we go through the motions of practicing the spiritual disciplines, but we remain empty. Identify how your purpose might be off course. Have you been lazy and neglectful? Have you been simply checking the disciplines off a to-do list? Have you been doing them out of obligation?

2. What areas of your spiritual life need a change of purpose?

Principle 4: Make a Plan

1. Identify specific areas on which you need to refocus in order to become spiritually healthy.

2. Write down at least one way you can begin to work on the areas you listed above. Set specific goals, such as "I will read my Bible at least thirty minutes every day" or "I will participate in corporate worship."

Principle 5: Create Boundaries

1. Whenever we neglect spiritual disciplines, we typically do so because we've failed to create some important personal boundaries that we agree to stay within. We may be spending too much time watching television, surfing around on the computer, or simply doing nothing. Set some boundaries for yourself. For example, "I won't watch television until I've read my Bible."

Principle 6: Find Authentic Relationships

1. Identify at least one person with whom you can share the plans you made in this section.

2. Write down a specific time and method by which you will share these plans with this person.

Second Opinion
Matt Carter, senior pastor,

the Austin Stone Community Church, Austin, Texas

A. M. M.: Do you see the current Western church as being ineffective in reaching people with the gospel and growing them? Why?

M. C.: Pastor Bob Roberts asked the question in a recent book, "If we (the church) could plant one thousand mega churches all over the United States over the next ten years, wouldn't we be able to completely change this country for the cause of Christ? The answer Pastor Roberts reached was, "No." Why? Because that is exactly what the church in the United States did over the last ten years. We planted over one thousand churches that have grown to more than two thousand members apiece; and yet, per capita, there are fewer people going to church today than ever before in the history of our country. Something is terribly wrong.

Why is this occurring? I think there are several reasons, but I'm personally convinced that one of the main reasons people in America are leaving the church in droves is because there is severe biblical malnourishment in the body of Christ. They're leaving in droves not because we aren't clever enough, not because we don't have enough resources, but because people come to church, are entertained, and then leave starving, anemic, and utterly ineffective for the kingdom of God. I believe this is a direct result of pastors not fulfilling primary responsibilities God designed for them through Scripture.

A. M. M.: What do you see as the primary responsibilities of pastors and church leaders?

M. C.: In Scripture, we see two primary responsibilities of the pastor: servants of Christ and stewards of the mysteries of God. The apostle Paul wrote, "Men ought to regard us [pastors] as servants of Christ and as those entrusted with the secret things of God. Now it is required that those who have been given a trust must prove faithful" (1 Corinthians 4:1 – 2). Unfortunately, so many pastors view themselves first and foremost not as servants of Christ, not as those responsible for stewarding the deep things of God to their people, but rather as servants of the church! I grew up in a church that expected the pastor to be available to meet the every whim and need of every congregant. If somebody was in the hospital, he better go! If someone needed to meet with him, he better be available! If he spent too much time on his sermon rather than with the people, it was said of him that he was "a good preacher" but "not a good pastor." Although hospital visitations, meetings, and coffee times with the church are important, Scripture reveals that they are not the pastor's primary responsibilities. Being a servant of Christ and a steward of the deep things of God are.

A. M. M.: Pastors and leaders easily assume the obligation for having to do everything for everyone, and so they neglect the necessary spiritual disciplines. What shift in thinking and pastoring is needed to mobilize the church to practice true biblical servanthood?

M. C.: The necessary shift for pastors is to come back to the primary responsibility that God intended for them. This is most clearly seen in Acts 6. After complaints had arisen within the early church that certain widows were not being taken care of (an important task, by the way!), church members went to the pastors and complained that their widows were being ignored. The response of the twelve apostles is fascinating: "It would not be right for us to neglect the ministry of the word of God in order to wait on tables. Brothers, choose seven men from among you who are known to be full of the Spirit and wisdom. We will turn this responsibility over to them and will give our attention to prayer and the ministry of the word" (Acts 6:2 – 4). So we can clearly see from Scripture that the primary responsibility of the pastor is the stewarding of the word of God so that the saints can do the work of ministry.

A. M. M.: How do you practice spiritual disciplines in your day-to-day life?

M. C.: I try to maximize the things that draw me nearer to Christ and minimize the things that sap my affection for him.

Chapter 14: Physical Health

When it comes to eating right and exercising, there is no "I'll start tomorrow." Tomorrow is disease.

— V. L. Allineare

Moderation is a terrible word to use when discussing things like exercise and lattes and dessert and fried chicken. The word wisdom is much more appropriate.

We have become a society plagued by terrible physical health. I honestly don't know how we live as long as we do (maybe it's all those preservatives!). We eat when we're not hungry. We seldom exercise. We are convinced we're caffeinated robots who can thrive on four hours of sleep a night.

And we're only lying to ourselves.

Eating healthy, exercising, and getting enough sleep are the three staples of physical health. Most likely I won't reveal anything new to you in this chapter. But obviously we're pretty terrible listeners when it comes to this stuff, so maybe the refresher course, as well as the encouragement to apply the five principles we've been learning, will jump-start us into becoming a much healthier generation.

Eating Healthy

Key Scripture

> Don't you know that you yourselves are God's temple and that God's Spirit lives in you? If anyone destroys God's temple, God will destroy him; for God's temple is sacred, and you are that temple.
>
> — 1 Corinthians 3:16 – 17

It's not just Americans who eat poorly. I was in Scotland for a few weeks, I tuned into the BBC show "You Are What You Eat." The host, Gillian McKeith, who is a nutrition researcher, visits families who are overweight or obese and gets to the bottom of why.

On the particular show we watched, a very large table was covered in sweets and junk food. Food was piled up everywhere — almost to the point of overflowing onto the floor.

I assumed it was what the entire family ate in an entire week, but much to my surprise, it was what the mother, all by herself, ate in a week. Later, Gillian asked the parents to scoop heaping amounts of sugar into bowls — the amount of sugar their children consumed in a typical week. It was the equivalent of several pounds of sugar.

Many of us have developed terrible eating habits. And these bad habits don't just affect us; they affect our children — and they'll affect their children too if we don't call a halt. Take a look at these statistics from the Wellness International Network regarding obesity in America.[1]

How Overweight Are We?

- 58 million people are overweight; 40 million are obese; 3 million are morbidly obese

- Eight out of ten people over twenty-five years old are overweight

Obesity-Related Diseases

- There has been a 76 percent increase in type II diabetes in adults thirty to forty years old since 1990

- 80 percent of type II diabetes is related to obesity

- 70 percent of cardiovascular disease is related to obesity

- 42 percent of breast and colon cancer is diagnosed among obese individuals

- 30 percent of gallbladder surgeries are related to obesity

- 26 percent of obese people have high blood pressure

So let me ask you this: Are you a statistic?

Time for some positive news. What happens when you eat broccoli instead of that bacon cheeseburger? Nutritionists say,

- You fight off diseases. By making wise eating choices, you provide your body with natural defenses against common contagious diseases such as colds and flu, and you also receive long-term benefits from cancer-fighting antioxidants and vitamins.

- You sleep better. Staying away from too much caffeine and other stimulants found in processed food allows your body to recognize when it's time to rest and helps you reach a deeper sleep.

- You lose weight. We've already talked about the harmful effects carrying extra pounds can inflict on you. Eating proper portions of healthy foods and drinking plenty of water help you lose weight.

Exercise

Key Scripture

> Physical training is of some value, but godliness has value for all things, holding promise for both the present life and the life to come.
>
> — 1 Timothy 4:8

I've read this verse several times before, actually thinking it dismissed the value of physical training. Let's take a look at the first part of that verse again.

> Physical training is of some value . . .

The New Testament frequently references athletic training as a discipline parallel to spiritual discipline.

> Do you not know that in a race all the runners run, but only one gets the prize? Run in such a way as to get the prize. Everyone who competes in the games goes into strict training. They do it to get a crown that will not last; but we do it to get a crown that will last forever. Therefore I do not run like a man running aimlessly; I do not fight like a man beating the air. No, I beat my body and make it my slave so that after I have preached to others, I myself will not be disqualified for the prize.
>
> — 1 Corinthians 9:24 – 27

> If anyone competes as an athlete, he does not receive the victor's crown unless he competes according to the rules.
>
> — 2 Timothy 2:5

Exercise is a discipline. My friend Spence is one person I admire in this area. Spence, like most of us, works a full-time job. I asked him to share his average weekly workout schedule:

SUNDAY: Run 4 to 5 miles or bike 25 to 30 miles before swim practice, which goes from 4:00 p.m. to 5:30 p.m.

MONDAY: 30 minutes on the elliptical trainer and about 20 minutes on circuit training machines. (Optional day off.)

TUESDAY: Run 30 minutes.

WEDNESDAY: Bike 25 to 30 miles or run 4 to 5 miles; swim practice from 6:30 p.m. to 8:00 p.m.

THURSDAY: 30 minutes on the elliptical trainer and about 20 minutes on circuit training machines, or 25 to 30 miles on the bike.

FRIDAY: 5:00 a.m. swim practice.

SATURDAY: Light running (2 to 3 miles) or leisurely ride on the bike. (Mostly to enjoy the Saturday morning. If I pushed too hard during the week, I'll take Saturday off.)

Looking at this schedule, you may think that Spence is a personal trainer or maybe just someone who's strangely obsessed with fitness. He's not. He's really just your ordinary, everyday guy who has learned the benefits of exercise. And now he loves sharing it with others. Here's his story:

About five years ago, I started to run to lose weight. At the same time, my marriage was going through some significant challenges. Little did I know that running would help me clear my head, work through ideas, gain energy, improve my overall attitude, and give me the strength to work through marriage issues. I could think, pray, and figure things out — all in thirty minutes of running for the day. The more stressful life got, the more I ran. It was my "me" time.

My marriage ended and my life completely turned upside down. Besides the support of friends and family and my relationship with Christ, the one constant I had was running. So I turned up the heat and ran even more. I began talking to a counselor, who wanted me to consider going on antidepressants. But at a following session, he noticed a change in my demeanor. He asked if there was anything I had done differently that week to cause the positive change, and the only thing I could think of was that I had increased my running. He told me to keep on running.

A couple of months later, I read an article in Runner's World magazine called "Get Some Running Therapy." It discussed the positive effects running has in combating depression, anxiety, and anger. A light went off in my head — no wonder I loved running so much! It was my medication to keep me balanced and on track with healing and growing.
I felt like God had put running in my life not only to get me through difficult times, but also to teach me the discipline of training for something. My stress level is very low, and the clarity I gain is more than I could ever hope for.

The Mayo Clinic lists four reasons why exercise is important in reducing stress (not to mention the overall physical benefits exercise produces).

1. It pumps up your endorphins. Physical activity helps to bump up the production of your brain's feel-good neurotransmitters, called endorphins. Although this function is often referred to as a runner's high, a rousing game of tennis or a nature hike can also contribute to this cause.

2. It helps you deal with your stressors. Exercise helps alleviate daily tensions and may also help you learn to better cope with your stressors.

3. It is meditation in movement. After a fast-paced game of racquetball or several laps in the pool, you'll often find that you've forgotten the day's dilemmas and irritations and concentrated only on your body's movements. As you begin to regularly shed your daily tensions through movement and physical activity, you may find that this focus on a single task and the resulting energy and optimism can help you remain calm and clear in everything you do.

4. It improves your mood. Regular exercise can increase self-confidence and lower the symptoms associated with mild depression and anxiety. This can ease your stress levels and give you a sense of command over your body and your life.[2]

As someone who struggles with depression and anxiety from time to time, I've realized the effect that exercise has on my mood. During one of these seasons, I reached out to Gary Kinnaman, a pastor and author who has written about battling depression in ministry.[3]

One of the first questions he asked me was if I had been exercising.

My response was, "No."

He kindly suggested I get off my "too busy" rump and hit the gym.

I knew better. And Gary was so right. Not only does exercise naturally help me get these chemicals a little more balanced, but it is also a great way to process events or frustrations. When I'm angry, I can pound it out on the pavement, music blaring in my ears. There are few things more cathartic.

I also think it's important to note how Paul finishes the passage I referenced earlier:

"No, I beat my body and make it my slave so that after I have preached to others, I myself will not be disqualified for the prize."

Recently, there have been several articles (some gracious, some not) frankly calling out pastors who talk about some sin from the pulpit but engage in a *very* gluttonous lifestyle with food and drink. It's an easy point of hypocrisy people can tangibly see.

Imagine Paul having this conversation.

"Hey Paul, you've been telling me about all this important stuff about the church and using analogies about races and stuff. But every time I see you, you're slamming a donut down your gullet and I can see the imprint on the couch where you always sit. I'm just not so sure..."

Aside from Biblical commands, Paul knew the importance of physical health in his culture. If he wanted to earn people's trust to spread the Gospel message, he needed to be consistent with *everything* so *nothing* could be called into question.

Sleep

Key Scripture

Unless the LORD builds the house,

its builders labor in vain.

Unless the LORD watches over the city,

the watchmen stand guard in vain.

In vain you rise early

and stay up late,

toiling for food to eat —
for he grants sleep to those he loves.

— Psalm 127:1 – 2

Sometimes our excitement and passion for what God is doing keep us up at night. I can certainly understand that. I've spent many sleepless nights, imagining what amazing things God could do in a situation or reflecting on something he was already doing. Other times, we lay awake at night wrestling with God, desperately crying out to him and pleading with him.

But I truly think these instances are special. I think they're exceptions to the rule. And in order to preserve their special character, I think they should continue to be exceptions.

Like the attitude we often have about not taking a vacation, many of us pride ourselves on not sleeping. We have so much to do and so much to think about that we stay up into the wee hours of the morning, convinced we can do more for God with less sleep.

I love what Psalm 127:1 – 2 says about working in our own strength instead of in God's. Cut-and-dried — if God's not doing the building, we're laboring in vain. If God isn't involved, even if we're rising early and staying up late toiling, our work is in vain.

There is absolutely nothing inherently wrong with work. There is nothing wrong with building houses (or churches or families or whatever it is you build). The Proverbs 31 woman is commended for her early rising ("she gets up while it is still dark"). Why is she commended rather than scolded for rising early to begin her day of toiling?

The Proverbs 31 woman clearly is working out of the overflow from her relationship with God. The other characteristics that define her (encouraging, wise, generous, strong, faithful, fearless, dignified) are brought to a conclusion in verse 30: "A woman who fears the LORD is to be praised."

One of the things that is easy to ignore is the fact that we are designed to rest. After working hard — physically, emotionally, spiritually, and relationally — we need rest! Otherwise, we don't just become tired; we become weary. And when we're weary, we have two choices: rely on God to refresh and renew us, or continue to operate in our own strength and burn ourselves out.

Several passages in Scripture encourage us to rest and to keep hope alive.

"Come to me, all you who are weary and burdened, and I will give you rest. Take my yoke upon you and learn from me, for I am gentle and humble in heart, and you will find rest for your souls. For my yoke is easy and my burden is light."

— Matthew 11:28 – 30

"I will refresh the weary and satisfy the faint" [these are the words of the Lord]. . . .

My sleep had been pleasant to me [this is a comment made by Jeremiah].

— Jeremiah 31:25, 26, notes added

Even youths grow tired and weary,

and young men stumble and fall;

but those who hope in the LORD

will renew their strength.

They will soar on wings like eagles;

they will run and not grow weary,

they will walk and not be faint.

— Isaiah 40:30 – 31

Even as we run, as we place our hope in God, we will not grow weary to the point of burning out.

And we can sleep. Without feeling guilty! Our sleep can be "pleasant"!

If you think you're immune from the medical problems caused by sleep deprivation, you are seriously mistaken. Here's a laundry list of potential problems.[4]

- aching muscles
- blurred vision
- clinical depression
- color blindness
- daytime drowsiness and naps
- decreased mental activity and concentration
- depersonalization and derealization
- weakened immune system
- dizziness
- dark circles under the eyes
- fainting
- general confusion
- hallucinations (visual and auditory)
- hand tremors
- headache
- hernia
- hyperactivity
- hypertension
- impatience
- irritability
- lucid dreaming (once sleep resumes)
- memory lapses or loss
- nausea
- nystagmus (rapid - involuntary rhythmic eye movement)
- psychosis
- pallor
- slowed reaction time
- slurred and/or nonsensical speech
- weight loss or gain
- severe yawning
- symptoms similar to attention-deficit/-hyperactivity disorder
- symptoms similar to - alcoholic intoxication

Developing good sleep habits will help you perform better over the long haul. Breaking the bad habits you may have formed over the last several years can be tough. Here are some tips that helped me go from tossing and turning to sleeping like a baby:

157

- Don't watch TV or get on the computer or phone at night. Some people think that TV or mindless Internet surfing helps them wind down before bed. Actually, it has the opposite effect. Did you know that the light produced from televisions and computers stimulates your mind? Your body was created to naturally associate light with alertness and dark with rest. If you stare at a glowing screen before heading to bed, you're provoking your mind to stay awake! Instead, try reading, meditating, or journaling before you doze off.

- Keep the same routine. Try to wake up and go to bed at the same time each night. Doing so reinforces your body's natural sleep rhythm. There's no such thing as "making up" sleep. If you stay up late, don't sleep in the next morning. Doing so will interrupt your sleep pattern.

- Keep your bedroom dark. The reasoning is similar to the TV and computer tip. The darker your bedroom, the deeper your rest. I'm very sensitive to any kind of light in my bedroom. Even the smallest bit of light sneaking in under the door will cause me to toss and turn all night long. Hang heavy curtains, turn your cell phone upside down (or leave it in another room), and set your alarm clock's light settings to the lowest possible. Put night-lights in your bathroom and hallways so you don't have to turn on the overhead lights if you need to get up in the middle of the night. You'll be able to fall back asleep more quickly.

- Relax. This one is hard for me. My mind is always going. I've found that keeping a notepad by my bed allows me to jot down any thoughts I might have or journal any worries I'm facing. By releasing them onto the paper, I'm helping to release them out of my mind. If you're struggling with anxiety at night, find a Scripture that assures you of God's faithfulness. I've used a paraphrase of Isaiah 26:3. As I lie in bed, I repeat over and over, "He keeps in perfect peace whose mind is stayed on him." And, though it sounds a little silly, sometimes counting backward from 1,000 helps me focus and relax. I don't think I've ever gotten lower than 900 without falling asleep.

- Watch what you drink. Cut back on the caffeine. It's common sense, really. Do I need to explain this? Doctors say caffeine after 3:00 p.m. is a common cause of insomnia. Even if you don't feel jittery, caffeine is still a stimulant that can keep your brain from entering your sleeping rhythm. And while alcohol may help you unwind or make you sleepy, you'll wake up before getting into your full sleep cycle.

- Talk to your doctor. If you've tried everything to get to sleep and you're still having issues, talk to your doctor. Some chemical imbalances can cause sleep deprivation, and only your doctor will be able to make a diagnosis. If you're comfortable taking medicine or natural supplements, perhaps you could try taking some sleep aids for a while. Valerian Root has been great for me. These can help you reestablish a healthy sleeping pattern. As you gradually decrease your dose, your body may be able to compensate and keep you there.[5]

Respond

Principle 1: Reconnect with your Savior

Using the space below or in your own journal, write a prayer or a poem or draw something that helps you understand that God has taken care of you. That it may be in our nature to hide, but it's in his nature to pursue you.

Principle 2: Own Up

1. Statistically, the three main areas we struggle with in terms of our physical health are eating poorly, not exercising enough, and not getting adequate sleep. Of the three issues, do you relate to one, two, or all three?

2. What are some specific things you have done to contribute to the current

state of each of these areas of your physical health?

- eating poorly
- not exercising enough
- not getting adequate sleep

3. Good or bad, do you accept your role in this?

Principle 3: Change Your Purpose

1. Maybe it's convenience that causes you to skip meals, eat fast food, not exercise, and not sleep. Maybe it's pride. Write down the underlying reason for your neglect of your physical health.

2. What areas of your physical life need a change of purpose?

Principle 4: Make a Plan

1. Identify specific areas in which you need to refocus in order to become physically healthy.

2. Write down at least five ways you can begin to work on the areas you listed above. Set specific goals such as, "I will exercise three times a week" or "I'll say no to the diet soda and yes to more water."

Principle 5: Create Boundaries

1. In ways similar to our neglect of spiritual disciplines, we often neglect our physical health because of a lack of personal boundaries that we agree to stay within. Set some boundaries for yourself in this area of physical health. For example, "I won't watch television until I've exercised" or "I'm taking

the TV out of the bedroom."

Principle 6: Find Authentic Relationships

1. Identify at least one person with whom you can share the plans you made in this section.

2. Write down a specific time and method by which you will share these plans with this person.

Second Opinion

Shawn Wood, pastor,

Freedom Church, Moncks Corner, SC

A. M. M.: How long have you been in ministry? And during that time, how much weight did you gain?

S. W.: The information on my driver's license (and the picture, for that matter) gives great testimony that I weighed in at a super-middleweight prize-fighting 168 pounds. Sixty birthday lunches, lots of "hey, check out the leftover cupcakes in the kitchen," and many, many "I'm going to Wendy's for some comfort food" days later I looked in the mirror and realized I either had to get a new license or lose about forty pounds. Losing forty pounds is much easier than dealing with the DMV and takes less time — so I chose to go for the weight loss.

A. M. M.: What do you think contributed to your weight gain?

S. W.: Busyness and lack of planning would be the main two. Honestly, I'm not under a lot of the stresses I've been under in previous church situations. I have great people on my team — we just get too busy. When we do, we start to forget that this whole thing is a marathon and not a sprint. I started to eat fast food a ton, graze in the office kitchen, and neglect exercise.

A. M. M.: Were there other symptoms that resulted from your weight gain?

S. W.: Emotionally, it was a slap in the face. I still thought of myself as the super-welterweight athlete who could run four miles in under twenty-eight minutes. Then I realized that, by all official standards, I was fat. Physically, I started having some stomach problems and was put on acid reflux meds, and all in all I was just plain tired all the time. I felt like I had run those four miles every night in my sleep. And as an added bonus for my wife, I began snoring — loudly apparently.

162

A. M. M.: What was it that caused you to realize you needed to make a lifestyle change?

S. W.: What really pushed me over the edge was applying to get a new life insurance policy. Because my cholesterol was "very high," I was put in a higher bracket for -"people of risk." When I realized that the insurance company thought I would die young, it scared the heck out of me. I had a new baby and a beautiful wife, and I didn't want to leave them. I chose them over Wendy's Baconator. I think it was a good trade.

A. M. M.: Over the course of three months, you lost forty-four pounds. How did you do it?

S. W.: My wife and I both decided to start eating right in January 2007. For the first three months of the year we ate "clean" — high-quality foods free of additives — and followed an extremely low-calorie diet. My cholesterol dropped seventy-seven points in three months, and we became an active family. In March of that year we added a gym membership, and we both still work out three to four times a week. I choose to make a date with the gym every Monday, Wednesday, and Friday at lunch — and my assistant knows I do not blow it off. I've found that the gym is much better for me than Taco Bell — who knew?

A. M. M.: How has developing and maintaining a healthy lifestyle contributed positively to your ministry?

S. W.: I have a ton more energy in the short run. My family life is just more active and more fulfilling as we have a ton more energy together. For the long run, I know, Lord willing, I'll be around to do ministry for years and years to come. Most of all though, and this may seem controversial, I did not do it for my ministry. I did it as an act of worship toward Jesus and as a sign of commitment to my family. If I take care of my relationship with Jesus and my relationship with my family, God will honor my ministry.

Chapter 15: Emotional Health

It's not stress that kills us; it is our reaction to it.

— Hans Selye

You can't see emotion. I guess you can see the physical response of what someone is feeling, but none of us possess the ability to truly see into someone's heart (or brain — or wherever it is emotion comes from).

For example, if you walked into the café where I'm writing this right now and saw me typing, you probably wouldn't think much of it. I'm tucked away in the corner, occasionally sipping some water and casually observing people as they come and go.

What you wouldn't see is my heart racing. One of my friends had to confront someone today about some serious stuff, and I just found out it didn't go well at all. I'm hurting for my friend and the person he had to confront and the tension that now dampens their relationship.

You also wouldn't see that I'm worried. That I know there are some decisions I need to make and that I'm afraid to make the wrong one.

Emotions can fuel our decisions — good or bad. If we're not open to guidance and solitude, we are susceptible to letting our emotions guide us and not the Spirit.

Depression and Anxiety

Key Scripture

I waited patiently for the LORD;

> he turned to me and heard my cry.

He lifted me out of the slimy pit,

> out of the mud and mire;

he set my feet on a rock

and gave me a firm place to stand.

He put a new song in my mouth,

a hymn of praise to our God.

Many will see and fear

and put their trust in the LORD.

— Psalm 40:1 – 3

Stress from our decisions and even from our environment can and will impact our emotional health.

When you're in a stressful situation, your body creates hormones — mainly adrenaline and cortisol. Adrenaline typically affects your heart rate and blood pressure, while cortisol affects your digestive system.

A by-product of cortisol is delivered to your nervous system as a sedative in times of stress (that's why after certain stressful events, you feel worn-out). Over time, this can cause you to feel depressed, anxious, and helpless.

Depression that is caused by stress hormones can turn even more dangerous, physically and emotionally. You can become sleep deprived (which we've already discussed), and if left untreated, sleep deprivation can actually cause some people to develop personality or behavioral disorders. To top it off, experts say that in some cases, the actual structure of brain cells can change when these stress hormones don't go away.

Some of the most faithful people in the Bible — the psalmists, for example — struggled with feelings of extreme depression and anxiety. There is a huge stigma attached to emotional problems such as depression and anxiety (which just happen to be two of the most common emotional health challenges). Sadly, this stigma seems to especially tint the views of other believers in the church world.

We aren't filled with "the joy of the Lord," so we feel guilty. We are plagued by panic attacks, so we think we lack faith.

We also feel extremely alone. We think if we reach out for help, we'll surely be judged.

David in Psalm 40 vividly describes his feelings, but he also recalls God's faithfulness to him. He declares that his posture is such that he "waited patiently for the LORD."

If you suffer from depression or anxiety, you must get help. Pastors, counselors, and medical doctors are all people who can assist you on your journey to understanding and coping with emotional health issues. The truth is, you can't do it alone. And the healing process will take time.

It is your responsibility to seek out the help you need. And God will be faithful. His timing is never late. And it's never early either.

Emotional Escapism

Key Scripture

> I hold fast to your statutes, O LORD;
>> do not let me be put to shame.
> I run in the path of your commands,
>> for you have set my heart free.
> Teach me, O LORD, to follow your decrees;
>> then I will keep them to the end.
>
> — Psalm 119:31 – 33

God has created us to be emotional beings. When we're hurting, we often think that changing our physical circumstances will fix our emotional response. That's when we get into creating unhealthy emotional escapes.

In the years following the time I was sexually abused (which was shortly after my family had left the church), I felt empty. At the time, I didn't fully understand all that had happened or that I had a traumatic experience. All I knew was that the pain and isolation I felt was indescribable. So I did what anyone would do — I escaped.

In the beginning, my escape was in the form of unhealthy relationships with men. I would do anything in order to be affirmed. I needed to feel worthy and loved. After a few years on that road, I realized I only felt emptier and more isolated. I started drinking alcohol. And when that wasn't enough, I would combine the alcohol with prescription anxiety medicine.

It numbed my pain all right, but it didn't allow me to work through it.

Over time, I stopped abusing the alcohol and medicine. My escape then turned into something a little less obviously sinful — but sinful nonetheless.

I became a workaholic.

Being productive became my escape. It covered up the emotions I still hadn't dealt with. It was in 2006 when, in a counseling session, my therapist started pulling the bits and pieces of my past out of my heart. And with it came a lot of pain. Pain I was hiding and allowing to build up over the last decade. Pain I didn't even realize existed. I was living with it for so long that it had just become part of who I was — and so I simply accepted it.

It was strange. My first instinct was to go find the biggest bottle of wine (OK, whiskey) and drink it until I didn't feel anything anymore. I hadn't felt that urge in a long time. I told my counselor this. And she helped me realize I was only trying to escape again. It was a completely natural reaction.

She wouldn't let me. Others around me who knew of the situation wouldn't let me. Over the course of a few months, I was able to face that pain. Feel it deeply, all over again. But I was able to work through it.

The key in escaping is *where* you run.

Do you run to something that only covers up your pain?

Something that allows you to hide in it?

Or do you run to God?

Do you escape to his healing power?

To his mercy?

To his grace?

If you're escaping from something right now in an unhealthy or immoral way, you may be a bit scared to talk about it with someone. What will happen to your ministry if you confess? You could be escaping into pornography (on TV, on the Internet, or through just dwelling on images in your head — you don't need a screen). You could be having an inappropriate relationship with someone — emotionally or physically, or both. You could be using alcohol or nicotine or drugs or abusing prescriptions as the place to which you run. Gaming? Gambling? Eating disorders?

Whatever it may be, you've got to stop escaping now. You may lose your ministry or your reputation. So what? Right now, it's a lie anyway. There is healing and grace in confession. There is power in truth.

The truth will set you free. And that's the only thing that will.

Respond

Principle 1: Reconnect with your Savior

Using the space below or in your own journal or in your own journal, write a prayer or a poem or draw something that helps you understand that God has taken care of you. That it may be in our nature to hide, but it's in his nature to pursue you.

Principle 2: Own Up

1. Sometimes the decisions you make affect your emotional health, and quite honestly, sometimes it has nothing to do with your decisions. However, you are responsible for getting help. Are you ready to be honest about your emotional condition?

2. Are you struggling with depression, anxiety, escapism, or something else that's contributing to your emotional burnout?

3. What are some specific things you have done to contribute to the current state of your emotional health?

4. Good or bad, do you accept your role in this?

Principle 3: Change Your Purpose

1. If you are suffering from an emotional disorder, describe what things are like for you right now.

2. How does where you'd like to be contrast with where you are right now?

3. What areas of your emotional life need a change of purpose?

Principle 4: Make a Plan

1. If you're not already seeking help for your emotional well-being, now is the time to begin. Identify the people who can help you begin to get healthy again. Circle any below whom you can seek out this week.

Pastor   Friend   Counselor

Doctor   Other _____

2. Set specific goals for your emotional health. For example, you may seek to talk to a counselor or pastor a set number of times per month, journal about your emotions, see a doctor and try a medication, or meditate on how to run toward Christ.

Principle 5: Create Boundaries

Setting boundaries can help us focus on where we need to grow in our emotional health. Are there any relationships that are causing undue stress and therefore really need to be addressed by you? Do you need to have boundaries to help you avoid unhealthy escapes? List below the boundaries and how they will keep you from choosing the way of escape.

Principle 6: Find Authentic Relationships

1. Identify at least one person with whom you can share the plans you made in this section.

2. Write down a specific time and method by which you will share these plans with this person.

Second Opinion

Gary Kinnaman, pastor and author,

Phoenix, Arizona

A. M. M.: You've thoroughly researched and openly discussed your experience with depression. What are some causes of depression?

G. K.: In our book *Understanding Depression and Finding Hope*, my coauthor Rich Jacobs, MD, and I demythologize depression, and we uncover two terrible myths. First, people commonly believe that antidepressants are mood-altering drugs. You know, pop a pill, and you'll feel fine in no time. Antidepressants don't work that way. Instead, they slowly "heal" a person's brain chemistry. If they were mood altering, you could buy them on the street! I can feel a half a glass of wine in my head in minutes. But an antidepressant? There's no buzz. I've taken 'em, and weeks later I'm still wondering if they're helping — until one day my wife says, "You've been so much easier to live with lately."

The second myth: Depression is caused by bad things happening in your life, like losing your job. Yes, everyone "feels" depressed when bad things happen. And when things get better, they feel better. Or maybe they were able to overcome their feelings of depression by getting their minds off their loss. Some have called this acute depression. In our book, we call it simple discouragement.

"Feeling down" is a common human experience, so we have difficulty understanding others who suffer from chronic or clinical depression, which is not essentially related to external circumstances. people who are chronically depressed can't just pull themselves out of it. Certainly, negative events can exacerbate clinical depression, but clinical depression is inside out — often the result of a chemical imbalance, the exact nature of which can be elusive.

A. M. M.: What first signaled to you that something wasn't right?

G. K.: I have a family history of depression, so the way I felt, as early as high school, just seemed "normal." For years, I lived with a residual darkness, especially when I got up in the morning, a mild form of chronic depression called dysthemia. I prayed. I fasted. I got prayed for. I got a health food store full of advice. I exercised. But in the morning, oh, I was heavy inside.

A. M. M.: Did suffering with depression change the way you did ministry?

G. K.: I don't think so. But it certainly changes one's perspective on God and ministry. All of us have some dysfunction — a euphemism for sin and fallenness — and anyone in ministry has to face their own "demons," be realistic about them, and let God's grace minister to them and through them.

It's like Peter after his denial: "After you've gone through this," Jesus said (and I paraphrase), "strengthen your brothers." How do you strengthen anyone after you've just had the worst night of your life? You realize you have nothing to offer but Christ in you. "We have a treasure in clay pots," Paul wrote. I realized long ago that I could not minister out of some kind of perpetual spiritual euphoria. I've had to learn how to serve God obediently and faithfully.

It has been said of Abraham Lincoln that, today, he would be declared unfit for public office. Yet, ironically, many believe it was his melancholy that empowered him, yes, empowered him, to lead the United States during the dark years of the Civil War. Lincoln, like no other in his time, was deeply empathetic with those who suffered on the battlefield, yet resolutely realistic about what had to be done to win the war. Shouldn't Christian leaders demonstrate these same qualities?

A. M. M.: people who are hurting often use escapes such as drugs, sex, or workaholic tendencies to cope with their pain. What are some healthy alternatives?

G. K.: In our book, Rich and I identify a number of practical approaches to treating depression. Among them are medication, therapy, Bible reading, prayer, self-talk, changing your thinking patterns, safe relationships, exercise, diet, even spiritual warfare at times. Depression is a comprehensive problem that requires holistic treatment.

A. M. M.: Many times, people feel alone or guilty because they have depression, anxiety, or other emotional illnesses. What would your advice to them be?

G. K.: I read recently — and I should have known this, given my two seminary degrees — that one of the original seven deadly sins was melancholy. Yeah, depression was considered a sin of the worst kind. Thankfully, the Catholic Church changed this a couple of hundred years ago when they replaced melancholy with sloth. Yet it's still not uncommon today to hear people say something like this: "Anyone who is persistently depressed is missing something in their relationship with God." Indeed, people have questioned Mother Teresa's salvation because, as she confessed, she felt distant from God and empty inside for most of her life.

To emote is human; to love those who emote is divine. Like some people who are better at baseball, or writing, or chemistry, some of us are just better — or worse — when it comes to emoting. Adam and Eve were naked and not ashamed. I've come to "accept" my depression as a part of the fallenness of my soul. And I am not ashamed. In many ways it's made me a deeper Christian and a better human being. I've heard the same voice that spoke to Paul: "My grace is sufficient for you." And it's made me less depressed!

Chapter 16: Relational Health

There's one sad truth in life I've found
While journeying east and west —
The only folks we really wound
Are those we love the best.
We flatter those we scarcely know,
We please the fleeting guest,
And deal full many a thoughtless blow
To those who love us best.

— Ella Wheeler Wilcox

When we burn out, our created instinct toward community also fizzles. In Genesis 1:26, God declared, "Let us make man in our image." We are designed for relationships.

Unnecessary Tensions in Relationships

Key Scripture

Better to live on a corner of the roof
than share a house with a quarrelsome wife.

— Proverbs 21:9

For some reason, this verse always makes me laugh. Maybe God's intent for painting such a vivid picture was to help us loosen up when we begin to take ourselves too seriously.

Stress and burnout can cause us to project our pain and exhaustion on others — usually on those closest to us. Some people respond to burnout by lashing out in anger — storming around in a rage as their lives are falling apart.

Exhaustion can cause us to shut down and stop communicating with our spouse or our friends. And by communicate, I mean both talking and listening. We no longer feel connected to those around us, and we begin to not care about nurturing those relationships God has placed in our lives.

After not communicating for a while, resentment can develop. Our spouses or friends may not feel comfortable opening up to us anymore, and bitterness can be formed and directed toward us, toward the church, and even toward God.

In Matthew 5:9, Jesus directs us to be "peacemakers" (in Greek, -eirəmnopoioi, from eirəmnəm which means "peace," and poieɑn which means "to do or to make"). It will take effort and intentionality on our part to bring balance back into our relationships. We are to make peace and strive for unity.

Inappropriate Relationships

Key Scripture

> "You have heard that it was said, 'Do not commit adultery.' But I tell you that anyone who looks at a woman lustfully has already committed adultery with her in his heart. If your right eye causes you to sin, gouge it out and throw it away. It is better for you to lose one part of your body than for your whole body to be thrown into hell. And if your right hand causes you to sin, cut it off and throw it away. It is better for you to lose one part of your body than for your whole body to go into hell."
>
> — Matthew 5:27 – 30

Burnout, in its most extreme cases, can push us to escape into inappropriate relationships.

Deep inside us, beyond anything we can comprehend, understand, or express, there is a need. This need presents itself differently, because we are unique individuals. For someone, it may be security; for others, it may be acceptance. Or affirmation.

Regardless of how these needs manifest in our lives, they all exist for the same reason. We need to feel loved. We need to be accepted. We need to feel worthy.

It's an ache nobody can fully verbalize. But you know what it feels like. It's emptiness. A burning. A resonating hollowness that resides so deep within your chest that you wonder how such a small space could accommodate such an infinite longing. It's like having all the air knocked out of you, but you continue to breathe in and out.

Looking at it logically, it should be easy enough to appease the desire this need places within us. I mean, if you believe the Bible, it pretty much sums it up in one verse in Philippians:

"My God will meet all your needs according to his glorious riches in Christ Jesus" (Philippians 4:19).

And if you throw in a spouse:

"The LORD God said, 'It is not good for the man to be alone. I will make a helper suitable for him'" (Genesis 2:18).

When you go through premarital counseling, one of the things counselors seem to be required to teach you is that your spouse is supposed to be your companion, and she is supposed to meet your needs. However, they always throw in the little disclaimer — "For those needs that aren't met, you should rely on God to meet them."

So sum it all up — and according to what we're taught, there shouldn't be a needy one among us. For those earthly desires, we have our companion and soul mate. And in case this falls through, God's a great safety net.

Right?

If only life were that simple. We are frail and fallible human beings.

It's not easy for Tim to meet my need for affirmation. Does he affirm me? Absolutely. More than I often give him credit for. But growing up without much affirmation, I know that the longer this need goes unmet, the harder it is to satisfy.

And when I'm burned-out, my defenses are down. If it weren't for the friends I have in my life, I could fall into a serious trap.

The power of this deep human need is probably one of the most compelling forces on this earth. I know I've let it run my life on more than one occasion. It has the potential to remove all sense of responsibility, of commitment, of reality. It releases your mind into a fantasyland where you feel completely fulfilled because you're valued.

Satan knows we're vulnerable in this area. And he'll throw anything in our path to tempt us. He will nudge us to feel worthless. He'll fuel a cycle of negative thoughts in our mind. And then he'll present us with opportunities to receive that validation elsewhere, which we can and should only find in Christ.

Emotional affairs.

> Physical affairs.

> > Codependency.

We must do everything we can to protect our relational integrity.

Isolation

Key Scripture

> The LORD God said, "It is not good for the man to be alone. I will make a helper suitable for him."
>
> — Genesis 2:18

When we burn out, we feel like we don't have anything to offer relationally. And sometimes, we don't even want to let people peek into our lives out of fear that they'll see the mess and run.

In 2004, the National Opinion Research Center conducted a survey in which it found that Americans are increasingly lonely and isolated. According to the survey, nearly 75 percent of people in 1985 reported they had a friend in whom they could confide, but only 50 percent in 2004 said they could count on such support. Lynn Smith-Lovin, a Duke University sociologist who helped evaluate the results of the survey, said, that increased professional responsibilities, including working two or more jobs to make ends meet, and long commutes leave many people too exhausted to seek social — as well as family — connections. "Maybe sitting around watching 'Desperate Housewives' . . . is what counts for family interaction,"[1]

I'm naturally an introvert and a bit shy as well. For me to go and seek out new relationships is challenging. But isolation isn't just unhealthy for us relationally. It also has a huge physiological impact. One study found that the magnitude of risk associated with social isolation is comparable with that of cigarette smoking and other major biomedical and psychosocial risk factors.[2]

We are made for each other. It may be difficult to step out of your isolation, but I pray that you will see God's faithfulness as he provides you with the relationships you need.

Respond

Principle 1: Reconnect with your Savior

Using the space below or in your own journal, write a prayer or a poem or draw something that helps you understand that God has taken care of you. That it may be in our nature to hide, but it's in his nature to pursue you.

Principle 2: Own Up

1. Are you isolating yourself from relationships? Are you having problems communicating in your marriage? Are you involved in an inappropriate

relationship? List the areas where you are relationally unhealthy.

2. What are some specific things you have done to contribute to the current state of your relational health?

3. Good or bad, do you accept your role in this?

Principle 3: Change Your Purpose

1. God has created us to be in community with others. If you are struggling in your relational health right now, why is that?

2. What areas of your relational life need a change of purpose?

Principle 4: Make a Plan

1. Do you have relationships you need to work on by becoming more available and participating socially, taking steps to improve communication in existing relationships, or ending relationships that aren't healthy?

2. Set specific goals for your relational health.

Principle 5: Create Boundaries

Not having enough time is one of the biggest reasons people become isolated or can't invest in relationships. What are some areas in your schedule that need adjusting in order to make time for more quality relationships?

Principle 6: Find Authentic Relationships

1. Identify at least one person with whom you can share the plans you made in this section.

2. Write down a specific time and method by which you will share these plans with this person.

Second Opinion

Brandi Wilson, pastor's wife,

Cross Point Community Church, Nashville, Tennessee

A. M. M.: What do you see as your greatest calling in being the wife of a pastor?

B. W.: I think my greatest calling is to encourage and support the staff. They are performing a daunting job that can consume a lot of their time, energy, and attention, and I feel called to "love on them" (such a Southern phrase). It might be as simple as an email letting them know that worship was great the previous Sunday. Or remembering to ask about a situation occurring in their family. I also want the staff member's family to know that we value them. We like to work on strengthening those relationships outside the walls of the church. We'll plan social events together, such as enjoying dinner together, hanging out at the pool, or grabbing ice cream after church. At Cross Point we put a huge emphasis on community, and I feel that my role is to help create and nurture that sense of community among the staff.

A. M. M.: As the church grew, how did your role change?

B. W.: My role as pastor's wife hasn't changed much as the church has grown. Thankfully, we've never served in a church that expects a typical pastor's wife, which works great for me because I'm allowed to define my role. That alone gives me the ability to serve in a ministry that aligns with my gifts and my passions rather than filling a spot because it is expected of me.

As Cross Point has grown, I've realized how much the congregation just wants to feel like they know our family. They'll attend a church of several thousand and know very few people, but they want to feel like they know us. They like to see that we're real people with real problems, facing the daily challenges that everyone else faces. People come to church looking for authenticity, and they love seeing that authenticity lived out in the pastor's family.

A. M. M.: What kinds of boundaries do you set to protect time alone with your husband?

B. W.: With three children we have a hard time being alone, but we guard our family time very carefully. What works for us is specifically setting time aside on the weekend for our family. That family time might be spent at home, at the ballpark, in the front yard, or even with friends, but it's definitely away from church activities (as much as we can control). Our weeks from Sunday to Thursday are usually jammed full of "life," and we both love knowing that we have some quality time coming on the weekend. Since we both thrive on being able to disconnect, we focus on weekends to reenergize us.

Another boundary that helps protect us is working hard not to "talk church" at home. We might discuss the surface stuff, but I know that when Pete, my husband, gets home, he has talked, thought, and worked church all day and just wants to be home — the place he knows is his refuge. So we usually discuss the "how was your day details" and then move on to life outside of Cross Point. I trust that if anything major is going on, he'll fill me in (it has taken a lot of practice for me not to drill him with questions, and I still fight it sometimes). Pete is encouraged by knowing he's not going to have to rehash his workday with me unless he chooses to revisit the day.

A. M. M.: What has been the most challenging part of public life and ministry for your family?

B. W.: The most challenging part is the expectations. Expectations go along with any job, but no one thinks pastor and then thinks "good time." People don't expect you to actually be someone they would enjoy hanging out with. They expect you to be stiff and full of rules. When people learn of Pete's occupation, we get varied responses. For instance, we've had neighbors who have built a privacy fence between our house and theirs, neighbors who have told us to never invite them to church, even neighbors who, after finding out that Pete worked for a church, have never waved hello again. But along with that, we've had neighbors Pete has baptized, neighbors we've been in community groups with, and even neighbors who say that Cross Point has helped to keep their family together. The good far outweighs the bad.

I do worry about how those expectations will affect my children. Being raised as PKs adds another level to the normal expectations of life. We're not going to allow other people to pressure our kids into fitting a certain mold.

A. M. M.: Why are relationships and community essential for you as a pastor's wife but also for believers in general?

B. W.: When someone asks me for my view of the best part of ministry, I always answer, "People" (they can be the worst part too). When I look back on our years in ministry, I always think about those special people who came alongside us as friends. We couldn't have made it this far by ourselves. We've needed those relationships to encourage us, support us, and remind us to keep our chins up. The thing I love about the way we do ministry is the fact that we don't do it to "bring home the bacon." What makes us do ministry — and love doing ministry — is the community. Cross Point isn't just our church, a place where we worship on Sunday. When we talk about Cross Point, it isn't a building; it's the community we do life with. It's the people we vacation with, the people we pray with, the people who call and ask about how our day went, the people who love our children, the people we can go to in times of trouble and in times of joy. They aren't just faces we see on Sundays, but people we come alongside and walk through life with.

Those relationships aren't just needed in ministry; they're needed in everyday life. I believe we are called to be committed to one another as believers in order to experience dynamic faith. Finding authentic relationships and a community that engages in biblical truth is life changing.

PART 5

CREATING A HEALTHY ENVIRONMENT

In addition to taking practical steps in our everyday lives, as leaders in ministry, we're charged with a unique responsibility to create healthy environments wherever we may be. If you're starting from scratch, this is a great place to develop values in order to prevent those in your care from burning out. But it's never too late to turn around and implement these, either.

When you go the hospital, you don't go to *get* sick. You go to heal. The environment of a hospital is conducive for health. The doctors and nurses are uniquely and thoroughly trained. If they're sick, they stay home. Everything is sanitary. Processes and procedures are in place to save lives.

So, what if you're not healthy? Does that mean you're excluded? Absolutely not. In fact, it reinforces the need for truly healthy environments to be solid and strong. A healthy environment would exist for you to join so you can begin to heal.

If you're sick, the rest of your body kicks it up a notch and compensates so you can heal. If your stomach is being attacked by an infection, your white blood cells increase in order to fight it off so you can be healthy again. In the same sense, if one part of the Body is not healthy, the rest of the body should surround it so healing occurs.

When I asked the community on my blog what they thought made up a healthy environment, I had a multitude of different answers. However, my friend Cindy left the simplest and most profound comment of them all.

Healthy people.

Healthy people make up healthy environments. You cant expect other people to do what you think should be done. You are responsible for cultivating healthy characteristics in your own life. When healthy people come together, a healthy environment is birthed.

We will discuss some characteristics that make people healthy and able to contribute to the overall health of a larger setting. All of the following four characteristics are transferable, meaning when a person integrates them into his or her daily living, it's inevitable the environment will be positively impacted.

Chapter 17: Characteristic One
Commits To Spiritual Disciplines And Common Goals

A healthy, Christ-honoring environment should be the number one priority. This happens by establishing a healthy hiring process, consistently communicating the importance of passionate and growing relationship with God, and ensuring the people you do hire are completely committed to the calling God has placed in front of your church.

Hiring

It's funny, but not in a good way. I recently went to a church staffing website to peruse requirements for ministry in modern churches. Here are some real results (Sorry if they're yours! Maybe this section can help!)

For pastoral positions:

Position 1:

- Bible College Degree

- Experience as an Associate Pastor or Better (better? What does that mean?)

Position 2:

- Seven or more years of pastoral experience

- Leadership experience at a medium sized church

- Ordained by a Protestant denomination

- Masters of Divinity degree or higher

For support positions:

Position 1:

- At least six years of professional experience in live event technology

- A minimum of an undergraduate degree in video production or a related field.

- Excellent computer knowledge, experience and proficiency with Final Cut Studio and Adobe Creative Suite.

- The ability to recruit, train and develop volunteers

Position 2:

- Excellent staff supervision and leadership development skills; as well as recruiting, time management, organizational, and judgment skills.

- Strength in verbal communication and writing.

- A passion for providing excellent customer service.

- Ability to work independently as well as to take direction.

- Experience in commercial rental and/or property management and event planning, including wedding coordination.

- A Bachelor's degree is required and an MBA preferred; other applicable graduate degree helpful. Certified Event Manager designation is desirable.

- The ability to lift 35 pounds

Now please, don't misunderstand. All of these traits are desirable for particular staff positions. And we need to know what our responsibilities are. What I noticed as I was browsing through open positions was only half of the ones listed had any kind of spiritual health requirements!

One would assume that people applying for positions at a church would automatically share the same values and relationship with Christ, but that isn't the case.

My friend Cory is a great example of this. He wasn't a believer when he applied for a Communications Director position at a church.

Cory writes,

> *After making some irresponsible choices, I decided I needed to get my life in order. And at the time, I was working for a magazine publisher that wasn't doing well financially and I was fearful of losing my job.*
>
> *A friend of mine, who unbeknownst to me, had been praying for my salvation, told me about a position at her church that was opening up. Apprehensive at first, I told her I'd like her to put my name in for consideration.*
>
> *I went to my first interview with an associate pastor. It was a good meeting and I felt like they would offer me the job as Communications Director. Later that night at home, I felt this strange sense that God had a plan for me to work there.*
>
> *A day or so later, the associate pastor called to say that the senior pastor wanted to talk to me. I was extremely nervous, because at the time, I could name only the first four books of the New Testament and hadn't been in church much for the last 5 or 6 years, except for weddings and funerals.*
>
> *At the second interview, the pastor wanted to know where I stood with the Lord. He presented the Gospel to me, and the key theme I hung on to was forgiveness granted through Jesus Christ. I knew (very much so) that I needed that forgiveness. So with the pastor, I prayed to*

receive Christ as my Lord and Savior.

> *It was an incredibly exciting and uneasy time for me. I was full of joy for having the assurance of heaven, but like a newborn baby in my faith, I was filled with thousands of questions.*

> *Serving on that church staff was so vital to my first steps as a follower of Jesus. I had every resource available to learn more about my God and godly, supportive people to walk with me through it all. It was all part of the path I believe God had been gently guiding me on."*

Cory's story certainly has a happy ending. Even though he applied for the position and didn't know Christ, those around him introduced him and they were able to disciple him.

Sometimes, however…you just don't know. Let's take a look at Jason's story.

Jason saw the ad for an accounts payable position online. He realized it was at a church, and figured it was probably time he started going back to church anyway. Surely the environment would be better than his current position at a collections agency.

He applied and interviewed with both the Finance Director and one of the executive pastors. The rest of the AP team went to lunch with him just to make sure there was team chemistry.

Everyone was under the impression Jason was a believer. Until his first week.

Lisa was one of the people in the finance department that trained Jason. As she gave him a tour of their rather large building, she couldn't help but notice he didn't seem to understand some of the basic terminology you'd find in an average church. He asked what words and phrases such as "ministry" and "children's service" meant. She gave him the benefit of the doubt. Maybe he was new in his faith and wasn't familiar with the "Christianese" so many of us throw around. However, Lisa was certain there was a problem when he didn't recognize the name Michael W. Smith.

Okay, she was a only a *little* worried he didn't know who Smitty was, but overall, she couldn't shake the feeling that it just didn't seem like Jason was comprehending the vision and mission of a church.

She talked to another staff member confidentially who promised to keep an eye out on Jason for a few weeks, just to see if he was picking up the same vibe. Sure enough, after a few weeks and several interactions, it was clear Jason did not have a personal relationship with Christ.

What do you do in a situation like that? Force Jesus on him? Don't say anything? It's a tricky place to be.

It seems so elementary and simple. If you're hiring for a ministry position, hire someone who shares the same commitment to Christ. Sometimes you have to spell it out.

Beyond that basic principle, a commitment to a *growing* relationship with Christ will be essential to making your team healthy.

Does this mean you need to only hire mature Christians for positions or only let those who have it "all figured out" have a role on your volunteer teams? Not at all. I wasn't the greatest example of a Christian when I started volunteering in a church. Sometimes the newest believers have the most passion and commitment to growing their relationship, and it certainly adds diversity to a team.

The bottom line? You must communicate the necessity of operating within the power of God. Skills are great. Education is nice. Even work ethic and attitude are key elements to ministry success. Above all of that, however, the practice of spiritual disciplines and daily depending on God is essential to both the individual's health, and the team's health.

If people begin to serve in any capacity in your ministry without realizing the importance of growing his or her relationship with Christ, you can expect them to burn out.

Committed to a Common Goal

A 2003 survey indicated at 25% yearly pastoral turnover rate. That means one out of every four pastors change jobs in a year. What contributes to such a high turnover?

I believe that it's the exact consumerist mindset that plagues church-hoppers, except we're the ones who fall victim to it.

Well, I don't like the way our finances are done. They don't give me enough authority to lead. They are never going to upgrade our technology. People say one thing and do another. There are so many politics. I never get any support.

I personally have struggled with the "Grass is Greener" syndrome. It's easy to look at the successes of the churches around you and be tempted to think that life would be so much better if you served at such-and-such church in such-and-such role. So, we become church-staff-hoppers.

We ask, "What's it in for me?" instead of "how can God use me here?"

And we jump ship to the next prettiest offer, only to find ourselves comparing and contrasting and complaining once again.

In order for your team to truly be healthy, the pieces of it must be committed to the unique call God has placed on your church. If you have someone who's only in it for kicks and grins, it has the potential to bring the whole team crashing to the ground.

Unfortunately, my friend Grant had to learn this lesson the hard way.

> *As a brand new church we have focused on making our worship services top notch since day one. Worship through music is a BIG part of what we do on the weekends, especially since we are in the Austin, TX area (Austin's the Live Music Capital of the World).*
>
> *After three years of incredible music we came to a point where we needed to hire a new worship leader. During that time, we got a call from a*

guy who had great musical talent and was highly recommended to us by a pastor at a church we admired. This young man had a family, seemed responsible, owned all of his own equipment, and was very well connected to our local music scene. We were excited about bringing him on board and were hopeful that he could meet our expectations.

After a couple of meetings with him, we hired him even though there were several "red flags" and reasons we shouldn't have. My gut said, "don't hire him" but my optimistic attitude and joy of finding someone let some of those warning signs slip by.

Over the course of the next year we quickly realized that our new hire was lacking in really critical areas. He couldn't lead and didn't care to. He didn't get involved in the church on any sort of personal level. This guy had a commitment to a paycheck; that was about it.

First we thought that we could help him and inspire him to succeed. We put into place some things that we needed to start doing anyway such as six-month staff reviews and staff retreats. We even gave the guy a pay raise. He began to meet our expectations on the performance side, but resisted teamwork and never stepped into the leadership role that we had hired him for.

As we pushed for a "Whatever It Takes" attitude on our team, he seemed to fall into a mode of "just getting the job done" with even less involvement in the overall life of the church.

His lack of initiative for development continued to increase. At a weekly team meeting, he surprised us by exploding with, "I'm outta here!" and a quick exit from the office. We were shocked.

After a week with little communication, he agreed to a final meeting where we asked for his resignation. He came with a letter in hand, ready to resign.

This hire wasn't just a bad thing for the guy that we had to let go; over *time it wore down our entire team. One wrong person on the team was causing mega burnout.*

We've learned a lot from this. Our plan is to move much slower when hiring in the future. Now, we know to look for leaders and people who are sold out to the what God is doing through us."

When someone invests into the call that God has placed on your church, there's no stopping them. They're inspired by what the future holds.

It's vital to the health of whatever team you are leading to clearly and consistently communicate that calling with your team. God has placed you there for a reason, and he's placed them under your care because he wants *all of you* to carry out this calling *together.*

Proverbs 29:18 says this,

"Where there is no vision, the people perish." (KJV)

Many times, the word "vision" in this verse has been misinterpreted to mean "goals" or "plans." The word "vision" in this verse actually means "divine guidance" or "revelation." And without divine guidance, people will perish. As important as it may be to be on the same page with your goals and your plans, without relying on God for wisdom and guidance that only he can provide, your environment will fall apart.

Without true guidance, we scatter. Our unity is broken. And Satan is one step closer to destroying us.

Chapter 18: Characteristic Two
Encourages Cohesive Relationships

Church work is hard. With so many battles being fought in the spiritual realms, we have to have each other's backs. Leaders are struck down in battle all the time, and it can be discouraging. From a senior pastor, a volunteer youth leader, a spouse, or a church janitor – we all have a Biblical mandate to build each other up.

In Judges 20, the Israelites fight the Benjamites (who had committed some pretty terrible offenses). After being sent into battle by the Lord (verse 18), they experience some alarming defeat.

"The Benjamites came out of Gibeah and cut down twenty-two thousand Israelites on the battlefield that day." (Judges 20:21)

WOW! They lost twenty-two thousand of their men. And God had sent them out? Instead of complaining about how God must be punishing them for something, they did something remarkable.

"But the men of Israel encouraged one another and again took up their positions where they had stationed themselves the first day." (Judges 20:22)

They encouraged one another! After so much bloodshed and discouragement, they challenged each other to get back up on the horse and continue the fight for justice.

Not only did they just encourage each other, they took their case to God. They were truly heartbroken over the loss, and they didn't hide it.

"The Israelites went up and wept before the LORD until evening, and they inquired of the LORD. They said, 'Shall we go up again to battle against the Benjamites, our brothers?'" (Judges 20:23)

God again confirmed they were to fight. So, on the second day, they went back up against the Benjamites.

Instead of handing them a clear victory, this time they loss eighteen thousand more men.

Ever had one of those days? The Isrealites were feeling pretty beat up at this point. I'm sure they wanted to give up. I'm sure thoughts of, "does God really know what He's doing?" crossed their minds.

But again, instead of waving the white flag, they banded together and demonstrated their camaraderie.

"Then the Israelites, *all the people*, went up to Bethel, and there they sat weeping before the LORD. They fasted that day until evening and presented burnt offerings and fellowship offerings to the LORD." (Judges 20:26 – emphasis mine).

All the people.

They united together and went to their Father, weeping. They fasted all day. They sacrificed burnt offerings (offerings that were made to demonstrate a complete dedication to God) and fellowship offerings (a voluntary act of thanksgiving and worship). Even though they had been so defeated, they were confident – together – and together expressed their mourning and hope through praise and thanksgiving.

They asked God one more time, "Should we go back and fight?" and God promised to deliver them. The next day, the Israelites sent the Benjamites running home.

Solomon said,

"A person standing alone can be attacked and defeated, but two can stand back-to-back and conquer."

In the movie *Gladiator*, Russell Crowe's character, Maximus, is faced with battling Rome's finest warriors to the death. Fighting alongside him is an entourage of foot soldiers. Maximus gathers them in a tight circle, back-to-back and shouts, "Stay together! Whatever comes out that gate, stay together!"

However, one gladiator gives in to the temptation to fight alone. He leaves the ring and is slain. Maximus knew they would be able to protect each other more effectively by staying as close as possible. And he was right.

Although our battles aren't against Amazonian warrior princesses, we are attacked from all sides constantly. Our marriages, families and integrity come under fire. Friends not only watch out for each other, they help each other defeat each and every adversary that enters the arena.

Sadly in churches, we're not just fighting opposing forces. We're also fighting each other. There is so much division in church leadership. So many politics, egos, and silos. Not only within the church as a whole, but even within our own local expressions of the Body.

We are broken. We are imperfect. But honestly? That doesn't mean we have to be jerks to one another.

A hurting world around us could care less whether we use hymnals or guitars or intelligent lights or pews. Only when they see our unity, our fellowship, and our support of one another will they truly see how the one true love that bonds us. When we fight, gossip, and tear each other down, we drag the name and the validity of a Saving Grace through the mud.

We have to present a light of unity to the world and we quite simply need to be a light to each other, too. If we don't, we'll be taken down.

Chapter 19: Characteristic Three
Thrives When Adapting

All living systems (that means us!) are dynamic; flexing and flowing as the environment allows. Most social environments (like work, church, and families) function as something known as Complex Adaptive Systems.

With the very simplest (and least scientific) definition of the concept, Complex Adaptive Systems have two unique characteristics.

One, they are complex in that they are diverse and made up of multiple interconnected elements. If you think of your church staff, ministry team, or even family, our individuality makes us diverse. From our age, to our experience, to our giftings, all of these things make us who we are (they're interconnected) yet they are typically unique.

Secondly, Complex Adaptive Systems are adaptive in that they have the capacity to change and learn from experience. If you've been in ministry for any amount of time, you realize the importance of flexibility. If your ability to go with the flow is limited, you will burn out fast! Also, in order to be healthy, one must be open to learning from mistakes (including your own and the mistakes of others)!

The theorists behind Complex Adaptive Systems have concluded that there are three stages these systems fall in. Environments are always changing, so if at one point, an environment is in one stage, it will eventually move into another stage.

The Adaptive Stage

The Adaptive Stage is the sweet spot for Complex Adaptive Systems (hence the name). In healthy environments, a majority of time will be spent in this stage. In the Adaptive Stage, freedom is king. Boundaries exist, but they are completely permeable. Diversity is highlighted, causing differences to challenge in positive ways. Communication is meaningful and trusted.

In the church world, this environment is ideal for the Spirit to move. We have our

199

limitations, but we are completely open to God's leading. Creativity is maximized and encouraged. The Body works together as individual parts. Much like what the Bible suggests in 1 Corinthians.

"There are different kinds of gifts, but the same Spirit. There are different kinds of service, but the same Lord. There are different kinds of working, but the same God works all of them in all men. Now to each one the manifestation of the Spirit is given for the common good. But in fact God has arranged the parts in the body, every one of them, just as he wanted them to be." (1 Corinthians 12:4 – 7; 18)

Organisms in the Adaptive Stage are moving towards a common goal: A cohesive outcome. If they successfully achieve it, they move into what's known as the Stable Stage, which allows them time for effective productivity (more on that later). If the organisms don't successfully achieve the goal because their unity falls to pieces, they then move into a third stage, the Chaos Stage.

The Stable Stage

Stability…it sounds nice, doesn't it? People are operating in the zone. Everything is balanced. People and processes are functioning properly. The Stable Stage isn't a bad place to be.

However, it's a bad place to stay. When left in the Stable Stage for too long, environments can become stale. Communication is made only from the top down without interaction from all members. People get in ruts!

How do I move from the Stable Stage back into the Adaptive Stage?

Remember, it's not a bad place to be for a season, as this is the stage from where most tangible productivity stems. But, if you've been in an environment for a while and you feel your passion is completely dried up or you're just spinning your wheels and going nowhere, it's quite possible your environment has been stuck in the Stable Stage for too long.

If you're a leader who can make immediate changes, start by getting some feedback from your team to confirm your inclination. If your team agrees, discover together what areas are most stale. Take your team outside of its normal environment – go to a café, a mall, an airport, a park – and begin brainstorming some new approaches to daily problems you need to solve. Remember, there are no dumb ideas!

If you're leading from a supporting role, now is a great opportunity to lead up. Write down some creative ideas that will help pull your team out of the rut. Talk to your supervisor or ministry leader and humbly make your suggestions.

I realize many of you in a supporting role might not be comfortable approaching your leader because you're nervous (and possibly, rightfully so) that he or she might take it the wrong way. If that's the case, try sharing your ideas with others on your team. If you're truly an island, share your thoughts with a close friend or your spouse and find a way to implement them in your own responsibilities. I promise changing your own outlook will positively impact the rest of your team.

The Chaotic Stage

As I mentioned previously, if in the Adaptive Stage, everything beings to fall apart, the environment will move into the Chaotic Stage.

The Chaotic Stage *is* as bad as it sounds. Let's look at some of its synonyms. Disintegration. Confusion. Anarchy. Pandemonium. Commotion. Disarray. Turmoil. Madness. It's random. There's no consistency.

Chaos is only productive because it helps us grow through pain. Through situations we would naturally avoid. When a body of believers enters this stage, those most willing to adapt emerge as leaders.

When my friend Allen's (the man from earlier in the book) affair was slowly made public, it was the epitome of the definition of chaos. Beforehand, when the church was in an Adaptive Stage, the body was moving to one common goal, reaching people for Christ and discipling them. When the pieces of the body stopped functioning properly (which happens in moments of unconfessed sin and unrepentant hearts), the fabric that bound the body together slowly started becoming unraveled. Over time, it unraveled into a state of spiritual inconsistency. At its climax, chaos occurred. Those who were spiritually in tune to the Spirit recognized the need for order.

How can we move out of the Chaotic Stage?

If you're in the midst of a chaotic environment, you'll know. Your team will lack the essential unity and organization. The right hand won't know what the left hand is doing, but in this case, that's not a good thing.

As a leader in a chaotic environment, *now is the time to act!* You've probably already been praying about the issues your team is facing. Please don't wait any longer. Sit down with the people you need to sit down with and make an organized plan of action now, including both short term and long-term solutions for protecting your church from entering in to the Chaotic Stage again.

Sometimes this may mean having to admit failure. And failure is okay. But when you do fail, fail *forward!* And share your failures openly and humbly. Others can learn from your mistakes.

Maybe you realize you are the agent that is causing chaos on your team. You could be living in unconfessed sin. Nobody's perfect, but we all must strive to keep our hearts clean and our spirits renewed. It's a process that must be repeated.

If you are that chaotic agent, you are grieving the Holy Spirit. Your sin is causing a breach in your personal relationship with God and quite possibly is affecting the other parts of the Body. 1 John 1:9 says this,

"If we confess our sins, he is faithful and just and will forgive us our sins and purify us from all unrighteousness."

Realize that this forgiveness and purification is conditional. You must confess. It's on your head. But keep the promise in mind when it gets scary and the courage is hard to find. *He will be faithful and just.*

Napoleon Bonaparte once said, ""The battlefield is a scene of constant chaos. The winner will be the one who controls that chaos, both his own and the enemies."

Some people live off the adrenaline a chaotic situation brings. It's exciting, and new, and challenging. But I think what we really crave is bringing order to the chaos.

Managing it.

Turning it into something beautiful.

...and something healthy.

Chapter 20: Characteristic Four
Communicates With Wisdom And Honesty

An admirable trend in recent generations is openness. Slowly we have started to reveal more and more of our struggles and our pains, but almost to the point where it's *not* healthy. Our focus has moved from the desire of our heart being authentic, to desiring pity for our weaknesses.

It's believed that open communication is a cornerstone of health. I'd like to take that a step further and say *wise* communication is a cornerstone of health.

Open communication says, "I'll tell you everything that's on my heart." There's no filter. We can forsake necessary empathy and tact when we are sharing *everything*. Wise communication looks at the situation and evaluates all of the elements.

What kind of environment am I in? Who are the people I'm talking to? How well do I know them?

Everyone we come in contact with is going to have a past, a present, and a future, just as we do. Wisely communicating with each other will save unnecessary tension and misunderstandings in the end.

Honest Listening

As believers, we have to be committed to honest interaction. Not just speaking honestly, but listening and processing in a spirit of truth as well. A piece of interacting honestly with others means is honestly listening. Honest listening means shutting off other activity in your mind. Like grocery lists. The football game. Your dissertation.

I struggle with honest listening because I've yet to master the art flipping the switch to "off" in my brain. At any given time, I can be thinking about a project at work, wondering if I forgot to feed my dog, remember I need to call a friend, pick up dry cleaning, and wondering what color shoes go best with the dress for my friend's wedding. Did I mention? All of this goes through my head while I'm on a date with my husband.

The two most important relationships in my life – my relationship with God and my relationship with my husband – deserve my *complete* focus. In addition to that, when God puts people in my life who need me to minster to, or people who he's placed in my path that I need to learn from, I am doing them a huge disservice by not devoting my attention to them.

"But Anne Marie, you really don't understand! I can't shut off my brain!"

Oh, no. I do understand that. Very deeply.

Many times my husband has heard, "Well, that's just the way God wired me."

The truth in the matter is you can shut off your brain. It takes work. Sometimes it takes *really hard* work. But it's possible.

The next time you're in a conversation with someone and you catch your mind drifting, stop it. Say to yourself, "I am going to focus on this person. God wants me to listen honestly." And then do it again.

And again.

And again.

Honest Processing

Honest processing is similar to honest listening in the sense you have to be focused on the person you're listening to. Honest processing is the next layer of the communication, when you take what you're hearing and you form judgments.

Let's take a look at a scenario that happened in a church I'm familiar with.

Monica is a full time church employee with a great attitude. She's a hard worker, consistent, and her co-workers love her. And she happened to fall and hurt her back. The doctor said she'd have to have surgery to fix her vertebrae. It wasn't life threatening, so she could wait. She returned back to work a few days later, and decided to gather some information on the benefits she has available. Because she wasn't sure how long she'd be out, she emailed her church's finance manager, who was the person responsible for handling benefits.

Robin-

I have an appointment scheduled with my doctor next week to discuss options regarding the timing of the surgery on my back. Do you know if we have short-term disability, and what I would need to do to qualify?

Thanks,

Monica

Robin, who had a tendency to over-dramatize things, immediately called Robin's boss, Daniel, who was the executive pastor.

"Did you know Monica is planning on having back surgery next week? She asked me about short-term benefits. She'll be out at least six weeks! I need more time to process this!"

Daniel was upset. He thanked Robin for letting him know, and walked downstairs to Monica's office. He closed the door and asked Monica if she had time to talk.

"Sure," Monica said, expecting nothing out of the ordinary. "Have a seat."

Daniel didn't sit down.

"Robin just called me and told me about your surgery next week." He raised his voice. "You cannot expect me to be happy about this! Not only did you not communicate directly with me, your supervisor, you go behind my back to turn in your paperwork to human resources. I am completely disappointed with you, and this mistake is completely inexcusable!"

Monica sat stunned.

Her voice shaking, she responded, "I'm not having surgery next week, Daniel. I only have an appointment with my doctor to discuss my options. I asked Robin about our benefits because I wanted to know what was available so I could arrange something down the road with my doctor. He said I'd be able to safely wait for a few months."

Daniel seemed a little stunned himself.

"Wow," he said. "I am so sorry, Monica. I didn't bother to check the facts first."

In this situation, both Robin and Daniel quickly jumped to conclusions. Robin didn't understand Monica's email and instead of attempting to clarify Monica's request directly, she went to Daniel.

Daniel didn't process Robin's phone call through his past experience, knowing she often overreacts.

Honest processing takes a situation and filters it through all known factors. Similar to wise communication, we must ask ourselves, "Based on the past, present, and future, how should I respond to this?"

If Daniel would have processed this situation knowing about Robin's personality and Monica's work ethic, he could have appropriately handled Robin's phone call and talk to Monica about her plans.

It's easy to form snap judgments, even when we don't have a history with someone based on appearances, positions, denominations, or associations. Honest processing handles incoming information with grace and in a light of humility.

Negative Feedback

For centuries, men have been tormented by eight words.

"Honey, does my butt look big in this?"

How *do* you answer that?

I recently posed a similar question to some friends (about how people respond to the question – I wasn't asking it!). Even though we were kidding around, the answers were all over the place. My favorite response was my friend Bryon. He said, "Realize that there is no way out. With confidence, fall down on the ground, grab your chest, and fake a heart attack!"

Christians are the best liars. Why? Because we do it in the spirit of love.

We don't want to hurt someone's feelings. We don't want to let people know what's really going on. So we tell people what we think they want to hear.

Christ did not call us to be people pleasers. Peacemakers, yes, but we can't sacrifice our integrity because we're worried about how someone will respond to truth. Speaking truth in love is essential to building the Body of Christ up into completeness.

Ephesians 4:15 – 16 states the importance of this.

"Instead, speaking the truth in love, we will in all things grow up into him who is the Head, that is, Christ. From him the whole body, joined and held together by every supporting ligament, grows and builds itself up in love, as each part does its work."

Before you do offer honest feedback that is critical and necessary, it is vitally important for your health and the health of the organization that you ask yourself a series of questions to make sure that love is your motivation for responding.

What's the condition of my heart right now? Could I possible be responding out of envy? Anger? Other people's expectations?

If you realize your own spirit is negative before you provide feedback, you may want to wait a little while. Process through why you're feeling the way you are. When your heart is ready to respond in the spirit of love, ask God to guide your words and your conversation.

Who am I responding to? Does he prefer to be directly communicated with? Is she more sensitive?

We must not only be aware of ourselves when we're providing constructive feedback. We must also be sensitive to the people we're with. Some people prefer a "don't beat around the bush" approach, while others may need to have a more personal interaction in order to feel comfortable and safe in receiving the feedback. If you spend too much personal time with a direct person, or if you're direct with someone who needs a little more attention, the conversation will potentially start on the wrong foot.

What kind of positive feedback can I offer too? Is there an affirming action step or an encouragement that I can contribute during the conversation or at the end of it?

This is an area I struggle with tremendously. Being a natural problem-solver and fairly direct in the way I approach issues, I have to consciously plan out ahead of time positive ways to influence the conversation. It's easy to say, "that graphic looks terrible," or "you were a little off key this weekend," and make a plan to fix the problem. Finding a helpful way you yourself can contribute to solving the problem requires a little more effort.

Positive Feedback

The problem we face with positive feedback is we don't offer it enough! I can't tell you how many conversations I've been in where someone has told me about a great job somebody did. Which is awesome! I love hearing about people's successes. Depending on the circumstance, sometimes I'll ask the person telling me if they've communicated that to the person who did the great job. More times than not, they haven't!

Maybe you're a senior pastor and you notice a greeter doing an outstanding job on the weekends. Telling that person's team leader so he or she can affirm the greeter is a good idea. But can you imagine the impact your words will have on him or her? You may not think it's such a big deal. You know you're "just a regular guy" like anyone else. But hearing the words come from your mouth will inspire and give so much confidence to that greeter!

If you see someone doing a great job, *tell them.* Just like bad news, it may come around to them second-hand. And praise is praise, even when it's second-hand. But hearing it directly is so much more meaningful and significant to the person you're complimenting.

Chapter 21: Processing through Pain

Why does it seem as though when another believer hurts us, the pain we experience is exponentially greater than if we are hurt by someone who doesn't share the same faith?

I wish I had the answer to that question, but I don't. All I know is that it's true, and the pain can be paralyzing. I wrote in the introduction that we weren't going to focus on the pain, but it is something that needs to be addressed. Now is the time.

In earlier chapters, I told a bit of my father's story and how being a preacher's kid affected me. Was I hurt? Did the actions of others cause pain to our family? More times than I could possibly write about.

But do I wish I had been protected from experiencing that pain?

Honestly, no.

One of the most frequently asked questions I get is from pastors concerned about protecting their families from seeing the brutality that often occurs in churches: "How can I protect my kids?"

And then they ask me, "What do you wish your parents had done differently?"

Not a darn thing. Seriously. I almost wish they had let me see more. I think it would have given me a healthier perspective — and a more realistic expectation — of what the dark side of the church can be like.

The most painful experience of my life happened during a time when I was in leadership at a church. My heart was severely wounded by a fellow staff member. Even years later as I write this, I have to be careful not to let bitterness creep back in.

What happened? Long story short, I opened up to a staff member. I shared my dreams, and he discounted them. I shared my weaknesses, and he exposed and exaggerated almost every one of them inappropriately to several other staff members. He lied and manipulated people on my team, sometimes plotting to turn us against each other. He set me, and others, up to fail.

It sounds like a movie, and a bad one at that, but it's all true. After being wounded, I wanted to throw in my ministry towel. Every reason I had for avoiding the church had been confirmed. I tried to remain involved in that church, but it was too painful.

Some of my dearest friends were involved in ministry there. They had questions about what happened, and in order to preserve some sort of unity, I wouldn't answer them specifically. I left. And that was painful too.

The process of healing from this experience is ongoing. It's taken several years so far, and I'm guessing it's something I'll always have to deal with from time to time. And if you've been hurt, you know the range of emotions you walk through.

Anger

Sadness

Loneliness

Doubt   Fear

It's almost impossible to trust again.

So, what happens now? Maybe you were hurt yesterday, or perhaps it was twenty years ago. I don't pretend to have all the answers. But I will share with you some parts of my own journey that God has certainly redeemed.

Preserving Unity

One of the mistakes a lot of people make when they've been hurt is to lash out. I made this mistake frequently. Once, I was literally trembling with anger after a meeting with the aforementioned staff member. As soon as it was over, I went into my friend's office and exploded, completely tearing my adversary apart. I trashed his leadership, his motives, and his authority. My friend, older and wiser than I am, calmly let me empty all my barrels.

212

After I tearfully finished, he shared an experience he had gone through at another church. He had been unjustly let go. But he and his wife decided to take the high road. They had plenty of opportunities to trash-talk their former church, but they refused to do so.

Before talking to my friend, I thought my only option was to lash out and expose this staff member for who he really was. The world needed to know. Or so I thought. But now, I was presented with the clear alternative — to keep quiet about the things that upset me, and move on.

It isn't easy to keep your mouth shut when someone unfairly betrays you. But except in rare occasions — when someone's health or immediate well-being is at stake, for example — it's necessary for the sake of unity.

Some of the greatest leaders I know have been severely hurt in ministry. I interviewed several for this book, and I discovered this consistent insight: the leaders who were the healthiest were the ones who never disrespected the people who hurt them.

Did they admit their hurt? Did they tell me their stories? Absolutely. But they also preserved unity. Being hurt is extremely painful. But we can't let our emotions dictate our actions.

Talking about It

Even though it's unwise to react emotionally and dishonor someone who has hurt you, it's extremely unhealthy not to discuss it. The key to doing this in an honoring manner is to find a mature and wise person who will look at the situation objectively.

What "talking about it" doesn't mean is fueling gossip with your friends. You may need to find someone outside of your church to talk to. My own process led me to get counseling at a faith-based counseling center on the other side of town.

Because my counselor was board certified, she was required by law to keep what I said confidential. It was an extremely safe place to unload, at times emotionally, about the pain. And since she was outside of the church's circle, her objectiveness encouraged me to look differently at facets of my situation.

One of the most striking things I learned by talking to an objective person was that the person who was hurting me was clearly also hurting as well. Recognizing this commonality somehow allowed me to see his humanity and brokenness instead of only the pain he caused me.

Praying about It

Working with a counselor also helped me pray for the person who was hurting me, which wasn't an easy task. But doing so was necessary for my growth.

Praying for this person was literally a life-changing experience. It not only helped me by taking the focus off myself but also brought me closer to the heart of God — which is exactly where I needed to be in order to truly love someone I considered an enemy.

Finding Strength to Forgive

For me, the hardest part of this process has been forgiveness. It's not a one-time decision. In a way, it's like marriage. It's a commitment you make for the rest of your life, because, chances are, you're going to remember significant pain indefinitely.

I wasn't sure how to forgive this man, but I knew it was something I had to do because I wanted to follow Jesus' example of ultimate forgiveness. I no longer wanted to be a slave to the negative emotions in my spirit. And choosing to forgive him meant abandoning the myths and learning the truth about forgiveness.

Forgiveness Myth #1: You Can Forgive and Forget

Many people think the phrase "forgive and forget" is an ancient proverb, rich with wisdom. Actually, it comes from Shakespeare's King Lear: "Pray you now, forget and forgive." Some offenses we're able to forget, but most of the time, there are things that can never be erased from our memories. Unfortunately, anything short of a lobotomy can't guarantee us the mental deletion of something that has hurt us. What's important is how we respond when these memories surface. Do we resort to bitterness and anger, or do we lean into our heavenly Father's arms and draw from his love to heal the wounds?

Forgiveness Myth #2: You Can't Forgive without Hearing "I'm Sorry"

One of the biggest issues I struggled with was the fact that I never received an apology. Whenever I would see my coworker at church after I had resigned from my position, he acted as though nothing was wrong, which only intensified my resentment toward him.

An apology never came, and assuming that he wasn't sorry for his actions made it difficult for me to even want to forgive him. Throughout the course of my healing, whenever I feel cheated, I reflect on a story that Jesus taught when asked about forgiveness.

A servant has become seriously indebted to his king — somewhere around the sum of $10,000,000. Moments before he, along with his family, are to be sold into slavery, he begs the king for another chance. Touched by his plea, the king releases him from his indebtedness.

After the pardoned servant leaves, he runs into a fellow servant — one who owes him only about $10. He immediately confronts him, demanding the money he's owed. The other servant isn't able to pay him back, so instead of pardoning the debt, the first servant throws his debtor into jail until he pays up.

The king finds out about the situation and is outraged: "Then the master called the servant in. 'You wicked servant,' he said. 'I canceled all that debt because you begged me to. Shouldn't you have had mercy on your fellow servant just as I had on you?' " (Matthew 18:32 – 33).

Yes, it is difficult to forgive someone who has hurt us, but I think of how many times I have been pardoned when I didn't deserve it. I think of how gracious others have been toward me, and how much Jesus sacrificed for my redemption.

By waiting for an apology that may never come, I was allowing this man's lack of action to control my decisions. To truly grow through this experience, I had to decide to forgive him, whether or not he ever asks for it. I have to extend to him the very grace that is extended to me.

Forgiveness Myth #3: Forgiveness Is a Feeling

After being hurt, it's natural to want to feel somewhat normal again. Instinctively, we want to do whatever we can to get rid of the pain and forget what happened. It's easy to deny the pain and try to hide it in the back of our minds. We occupy ourselves with activities or other relationships in order to avoid feeling the heartache. Or maybe we numb the pain by abusing alcohol or drugs.

I initially allowed my feelings to hold me back from forgiving my coworker who hurt me. I decided I wasn't ready to forgive him. In the midst of the pain I continued to feel, I convinced myself that when the time was right, I would know it, because I would be emotionally able to let it go.

However, after being hurt, we may never feel ready to forgive someone. When forgiveness is necessary, it means that someone has caused us pain. Forgiveness is deciding to move on in spite of our emotions. The more quickly we can begin the process of forgiveness, the less control we allow our pain to have in our lives.

Jesus set a consistent example of forgiving quickly. He said to the paralyzed man, "Take heart, son; your sins are forgiven" (Matthew 9:2), without the man even asking for forgiveness. As he was hanging on a cross, Jesus forgave those who crucified him without them seeking it: "Father, forgive them, for they do not know what they are doing" (Luke 23:34).

Our heavenly Father knows us intricately — inside and out. He knitted together the very fibers of our being, including our spirit. He wants nothing more than to be close to us. He knows that when we refuse to forgive, the bitterness that results will saturate our soul. As time passes, we begin to lose the ability to recognize his gentle touches in our lives. Before long, we isolate ourselves from the only One who will never bring us harm.

Throughout Scripture, we find example after example of forgiveness. God knew it wouldn't be easy for us to forgive, and he offers us the courage we need to extend forgiveness and the strength we need to heal. It's up to us to take the first step and begin the journey of forgiveness.

Trusting Again

One of the most difficult parts of this process has been finding the courage to trust again. I truly believed I could trust this staff person when I opened up to him. After all, he had encouraged me to talk to him about my goals. He was the one who wanted to hear my hopes and dreams for ministry, and he had the authority to help catapult them forward.

One of the passions I shared with him was forming a supportive community for artists — musicians, writers, painters, sculptors, whatever-ers. If it was art to you, it was art to me. The community I lived in at the time didn't have much to offer artists. So I had a dream to open a gallery and café within our church. We had the space to do it — and the money as well.

After sharing my idea with this person, he gave me the OK to pursue it completely, as long as it didn't interfere with my daily responsibilities. I spent countless nights drawing out plans, writing a proposal and a mission statement. I connected with local musicians and artists, and I spread the vision everywhere I went. I also helped design the room, from picking out colors to visiting other galleries to evaluating lighting options.

One day, the staff member pulled me aside to ask how I thought the process was going. Elated, I told him everything I had been doing. He asked me if I'd like to manage it when it opened up. "Are you kidding me? Yes!" I responded.

He asked me some practical questions too. Did I have any experience as a barista? No, but I could learn. What about experience in retail — did I have any? Right after high school, I managed a Christian bookstore and loved it. I knew how to inventory and clean and report and manage teams. Plus, we had a ton of passionate volunteers who were willing to chip in.

Then he asked me the million-dollar question:

Would you rather manage the gallery or stay in your current position?

I didn't have to think very long. I had already been thinking about it. I had been praying about it. I had even talked to some friends about it. "If it was going to be a full-time position, I'd love to transition over and take it on," was what I told him.

That answer gave him all the ammunition he needed to shoot that dream right between the eyes.

"What would you do if I didn't let you manage the gallery? Would you quit?"

I was totally confused.

"No. I would continue in what I'm currently doing. If you didn't think I was going to be the right person for that job, I'd trust you'd find the right person. I just want it to be successful, and I can certainly help as a volunteer if I need to."

"Well, it's obvious your heart is not in your current job. It's in this gallery. And I don't think you have the experience to run it. So I'm not going to offer it to you. I think you might want to consider your future on our staff."

Blindsided.

Are you kidding me?

I wasn't surprised by the fact that he wasn't offering me the job, although it appeared to have been his initial intent in our meeting. I was completely shocked that he had set me up. I told him I would make sure I'd keep doing a good job in my current position, and I left the meeting before I began bawling in front of him.

From this point on, life as I knew it on this church staff would never be the same. He began telling other staff members that I was performing poorly (even though my review from a few weeks prior had exceeded expectations in almost every area). He changed my schedule, which made it difficult to work with the team members I needed to work with. One of the final straws was when he forcefully took over a major project I was responsible for. Even though it was moving along successfully and had the approval of each of the key staff leaders, he verbally declared in a public meeting he was "pulling rank and taking over."

My confidence sunk. Maybe I was a terrible performer. Maybe I wasn't capable of handling minor decisions. Maybe the gallery idea was stupid.

Even I started believing the lies.

So a short time after he took over the project, I "resigned." (You know how that works – I made it back to my office after another heated meeting and emailed off my resignation letter before he could have me terminated).

I may have left my post on staff, but I never stopped believing those lies.

I was terrified to return to ministry. Honestly, I was terrified to return to any kind of job. I questioned my ministry calling. I questioned my leadership capabilities. I questioned my faith.

Over the last several years, I've found it difficult to share my biggest dreams and passions with people. I'm afraid that if I reveal my innermost thoughts, somehow they'll be used against me.

I recently was at a tech conference, and one of my favorite career writers, Penelope Trunk, shared some thoughts on life and career. She said something I believe is so true.

"People are afraid to be amazing."

I almost broke down crying right then and there.

Right now? I'm still hurting from that painful experience. I'm afraid to be amazing because I'm afraid to trust again. I know that I haven't yet fully regained the confidence I had several years ago. And I know it's stopping me from allowing God to work in me — for his greatness.

Remember, Satan will do anything to beat us down and make us ineffective for the kingdom. This includes warping our perspective on trusting others and ourselves again.

Trusting God

One of the first steps in learning to trust again is realizing that unless we fully trust God and his sovereignty, it will be impossible to trust others. The psalmist writes:

> [A righteous person] will have no fear of bad news;
>
>> his heart is steadfast, trusting in the LORD.
>
> — Psalm 112:7

When someone betrays your trust, it crushes your heart. The Hebrew word translated "steadfast" is kûn, which means "to be erect, to set up — certain (-ty) confirm, direct, faithfulness, be fixed, be stable."[1] We are promised that when we trust the Lord, our hearts become capable of being fixed and stable — even in those times when we face difficult circumstances.

If you've been hurt and are processing through a time of healing, ask yourself if you are trusting God. If you're not, read through the book of Psalms. You'll find many verses that will remind you of God's faithfulness.[2] He can be trusted.

Trusting Others

Trusting others is similar to forgiving others in the sense that it's a conscious decision, not a feeling. It involves a willful effort.

Some think that it takes two to dance the dance of trust.

> That trust must be earned.

> That people must be proven trustworthy over time.

While there is some truth to this (you wouldn't trust a convicted child molester to babysit for you), the Bible talks about trust in a different light. The apostle Paul writes, "[Love] . . . always trusts" (1 Corinthians13:7). The kind of love he writes about here is agapæn love — a sacrificial love that places the needs of others above yourself. You have to be reckless in the way you love, even after you're hurt. And even if you are hurt again.

Learning to Trust Fearlessly

We will continue to experience pain and hurt in life. We'll continue to be betrayed. The truth is, humans are just what they are — human. We make mistakes. You'll be let down, and you will also let down. The key is to trust fearlessly.

How can we trust fearlessly? By knowing that God is protecting us.

Always.

And the enemy is out to destroy us.

Always.

When you are tempted to give up on trust, remember truth.

God wants you to dream again.

God wants you to trust again.

Jesus came to give you life.

An abundant life.

God offers you a life not lacking in anything — including trust.

Epilogue: Resting in Abundant Life

As I mentioned earlier, I took a trip to Uganda with Compassion International. It was the most difficult and rewarding experience of my life so far. Our group arrived at 12:30 a.m., and after traveling for almost thirty hours, I was able to sleep a couple of hours before heading out with the team to visit a variety of child-development projects, meet church leaders, and play with children living in poverty.

The trip became more and more intense as the days went on. We visited a project focused on child survival. We made formula of diluted milk, olive oil, and grain for babies. We hugged teenage mothers and carried around toddlers. The next day, we visited one of the only HIV/AIDS-focused hospitals in the world. Children ran and played, oblivious to their imminent fate (something that haunted us all); the ones closest to death lay still in beds in open-air rooms, their atrophied arms pierced by life-giving needles and fluids.

With each day, our unusually extroverted group grew more solemn. And our trip leaders knew that this kind of reaction would happen. With little sleep, lots of spiritual warfare, and the contrast of death and hope, poverty and richness, and war and love surrounding us, they knew we would need to decompress.

They knew we would need to rest.

After three solid days of intense experiences, we took a small plane (an intense experience in and of itself) to a spot about 250 miles away from Kampala, the country's largest city. A generator powered the lodge at which we were staying. The nearest medical facility was six hours away on unpaved and potentially unsafe roads.

We were in the middle of nowhere.

And it was time to rest.

One afternoon, we took a ferry across the Nile River and then hopped into a small bus. We drove for a half hour on the bumpiest dirt road one could imagine before coming to Murchison Falls, one of the many wonders of the world. We then hiked another half hour to the very top.

Slowly we progressed on a narrow, rocky trail, dodging tree branches and mosquitoes along the way. We occasionally stopped at the most beautiful parts of the rapids, taking pictures of each other, but for the most part, the hike remained the quietest part of the trip.

As we reached the top of the falls, we passed several signs warning us of the steep cliffs and the danger that waited. Nobody was scared. Everyone was in awe. We helped each other over the slippery rocks and finally reached the very top.

They say many people have died at Murchison Falls. There are no railings to stop you from falling over. It's you, the rocks, and the falls. The beauty of water is transformed into something breathtaking. People become mesmerized by the unique blend of tranquility and power. Standing as close to the edge as our leaders and guides would let us, we let the wind-carried spray slowly drench us. Any fears of falling, of accidentally swallowing unclean water, of getting ravished by malaria-carrying mosquitoes — those fears had all vanished.

The hardships of the trip — the pain we saw, the poverty, and the brokenness — those things didn't disappear or float away in the rapids of the Nile. But taking a day to rest — to go to a quiet place and be reminded of the incredible power of the Creator — made me fall even more in awe of his sovereignty and his ultimate message of hope.

Rest bound together the incomplete to the complete.

We were refreshed. Inspired. Re-created. And we were able to rest in the knowledge and grace that, although there are many things for us to do, we are already a part of "on earth as it is in heaven."

Rest.

It is that simple command.

Humble.

Concerned.

Wise.

Loving.

"Come with me by yourselves to a quiet place and get some rest."

And rest, knowing that the work is already made complete by a cross, and that you belong to a Savior who wants nothing more for you than to live a fully abundant life.

It's your turn.

Go with him. Alone.

To a quiet place.

And rest.

Notes

Chapter 2: Comparing Mad Cow Disease to Mad Church Disease

1. See Centers for Disease Control and Prevention, "BSE (Bovine Spongiform Encephalopathy, or Mad Cow Disease)," http://www.cdc.gov/ ncidod/dvrd/bse/.

Chapter 3: The Emergency

1. Ellison Research, "Exclusive Findings from Ellison Research," http://www.ellisonresearch.com/PublicStudies.htm.

2. Apollo Health online, "Sleep Statistics," http://www.apollolight.com/sleep_stats.html.

3. Ellison Research, "Just How Healthy Is the Typical Pastor?" http://www.ellisonresearch.com/releases/20030801.htm.

4. Ibid.

5. Craig Groeschel, "Lessons from My Kids 2 (of 5)," http://swerve.lifechurch.tv/2007/10/page/2/.

6. Ellison Research, "New Research Shows Pastors May Not Have a Realistic View of the Health of Their Own Family," http://www.ellisonresearch.com/ERPS%20II/release_17_family.htm.

7. Thanks, Wes Hamilton, for calling attention to this book on your Facebook. Please read this book with caution. You can view *Preacher and Prayer* online at http://www.thecorner-stone.org/preacher_prayer_1.html.

8. See Ellison Research, "Study Shows Only 16% of Protestant Ministers Are Very Satisfied with Their Personal Prayer Lives," http://www. ellisonresearch.com/ERPS%20II/release_16_prayer.htm.

9. Excerpt from Bounds, *Preacher and Prayer*, chapter 1, http://www.thecorner-stone.org/preacher_prayer_1.html.

Chapter 4: Internal Risk Factors

1. See Meyer Friedman and Ray H. Rosenman, Type A Behavior and Your Heart (New York: Knopf, 1974).

Chapter 6: Symptoms

1. Archibald Hart, "Depressed, Stressed, and Burned Out: What's Going On in My Life?" Enrichment Journal, http://enrichmentjournal.ag.org/200603/200603_020_burnout.cfm.

Part 3: Getting Healthy: Six Principles of Recovery

1. W. E. Vine, *Vine's Complete Expository Dictionary of Old and New Testament Words* (Nashville: Nelson, 1996), 525.

Chapter 13: Spiritual Health

1. For a very helpful framework, see the discussion on the discipline of service in Richard Foster, *Celebration of Discipline* (New York: Harper & Row, 1978), 111 – 13. The comparisons in the chart are adapted from Foster's book.

Chapter 14: Physical Health

1. Wellness International Network, "Obesity Statistics," http://web.winltd.com/Article.aspx?PageURL=/Pages/English/healthnews/obesitystats.htm.

2. Mayo Clinic, "Exercise: Rev Up Your Routine to Reduce Stress," http://www.mayoclinic.com/health/exercise-and-stress/SR00036.

3. Gary Kinnaman and Richard Jacobs, *Seeing in the Dark: Getting the Facts on Depression and Finding Hope Again* (Minneapolis: Bethany, 2006).

4. See Wikipedia, "Sleep Deprivation,"

http://en.wikipedia.org/wiki/Sleep_deprivation.

5. For helpful information about sleep issues, see Better Health Channel, "Fact Sheet: Sleep Deprivation," http://www.betterhealth.vic.gov.au/bhcv2/bhcpdf.nsf/ByPDF/Sleep_deprivation/$ File/Sleep_deprivation.pdf ; Postgraduate Medicine Online, "Patient Notes: Sleep Deprivation," http://www.postgradmed.com/issues/2002/10_02/pn_sleep.shtml; Franklin Institute Online, "The Human Brain: Sleep and Stress," http://www.fi.edu/learn/brain/sleep.html.

Chapter 16: Relational Health

1. Shankar Vedantam, "Social Isolation Growing in U.S., Study Says," http://www.washingtonpost.com/wp-dyn/content/article/2006/06/22/AR2006062201763_pf.html.

2. See James S. House, "Social Isolation Kills, But How and Why?" Psychosomatic Medicine 63 (2001): 273 – 74, http://www.psychosomaticmedicine.org/cgi/content/full/63/2/273#R1-087713.

Chapter 20: Processing through Pain

1. James Strong, *The New Strong's Complete Dictionary of Bible Words* (Nashville: Nelson, 1996), #3559, p. 401.

2. Here are some places to begin: Psalm 9:10; 22:4 – 5; 32:10; 37:3 – 6; 91; 118:6 – 9; 125:1 – 2.

3. Watchman Nee, *Sit, Walk, Stand* (Downers Grove, Ill.: Tyndale, 1977), 16.

4. For a good overview, see the online article "The Sabbath Rest," http://www.gospel-herald.com/sabbath_studies/sabbath_rest.htm.

5. Nee, *Sit, Walk, Stand*, 16.

Acknowledgments

Tim, you deserve more than a thank you in a book. Through you, God has redeemed the most broken stories in my life.

To my family, I can't thank you enough for always supporting me regardless of how outlandish my dreams have been and for giving me a hand when those dreams have gotten me in trouble. Your courage in ministry has shown me that the beauty of the church is something worth fighting for.

In the last several years of ministry, I have been blessed and honored to have so many amazing people cross my path. It would be impossible to list everyone, so I do ask for your grace if I don't mention you, and I hope I've expressed my gratitude to you before.

Several gracious leaders contributed to this book with their wisdom and insight, and others boldly shared stories with me. Thank you for letting the world into your life, your pain, and your hope.

The Rest of God, Mark Buchanan's incredible book on Sabbath rest, has reshaped the way I think about rest, and I highly recommend that you read it.

And last, but certainly not least — to every person who has ever been a part of the community on my blog, who has supported this book during this long and amazing process: the words "thank you" do not express the depth of my appreciation. With your stories and your encouragement, this book has come to life.

About the Author

For more on Anne Marie Miller or to purchase resources and books, visit her website online at AnneMarieMiller.com.

CPSIA information can be obtained at www.ICGtesting.com
Printed in the USA
LVOW11s2230070115

421897LV00005B/335/P